Acclaim for

HOW TO NOURISH YOURSELF THROU

"Sterling and Crosbie's new book is a wonderful, detailed, medically sound, and super-helpful resource for adults working through recovery from an eating disorder. Offering an alternative to counting and tallying nutritional practices, this comprehensive and inclusive book offers start-today strategies and long-term support."

—**Jennifer L. Gaudiani, MD, CEDS-S, FAED,** founder and medical director of Gaudiani Clinic and author of *Sick Enough*

"This book is an essential starting point—and easy-to-follow guide—for anyone struggling with disordered eating or body image. It provides not just an accessible, evidence-based path to recovery, but also promotes a sense of balance and autonomy."

—**Norman Kim, PhD,** Center for Practice Innovations at Columbia University Department of Psychiatry

"This book is a wonderful, much-needed resource that simplifies and demystifies the nutrition process for those in recovery from an eating disorder and anyone who cares for them. Professionals and individuals will find themselves referring back to this book time and again. I look forward to sharing this as a resource with professionals, clients, and support system members alike!"

—**Christyna Johnson, MS, RDN, LDN**

"Filled with practical strategies and applications to help adults navigate the nutritional complexities of eating disorder recovery, this book will provide hope and guidance to those seeking greater joy and freedom with food, body, and movement."

—**Riley Nickols, PhD, CEDS-S,** counseling and sport psychologist and founder of Mind Body Endurance

"Having adopted the Plate-by-Plate Approach® as my foremost recommendation for parents of my adolescent clients grappling with eating disorders, I eagerly awaited this new book tailored to adults. This book provides a clear, compassionate, and all-encompassing framework applicable to all adults across the spectrum of eating issues, no matter their age, cultural background, and gender orientation. I wholeheartedly recommend this book to anyone questioning the healthfulness of their relationship to food and looking for a validating, encouraging guide toward healing."

—**Natalie Rose Allen, MPsy, RP,** eating disorder therapist

"This book is an invaluable resource. With a compassionate approach grounded in science, Sterling and Crosbie expertly support those striving to nourish themselves through an eating disorder."

—**Shelley Aggarwal, MD,** coauthor of *No Weigh!*

"Wendy and Casey have done it again! In adapting the Plate-by-Plate Approach® for adults, this book will provide much-needed support for both community and health professionals. This is going straight to the top of my recommendations list."

—**Fiona Sutherland, MSc, APD, CEDC,** The Mindful Dietitian

How to Nourish Yourself Through an Eating Disorder

Also by Wendy Sterling and Casey Crosbie

How to Nourish Your Child Through an Eating Disorder

How to Nourish Yourself Through an Eating Disorder

Recovery for Adults with the Plate-by-Plate Approach®

Wendy Sterling, MS, RD, CSSD, CEDS-S
Casey Crosbie, RD, CEDS-S

THE EXPERIMENT

NEW YORK

HOW TO NOURISH YOURSELF THROUGH AN EATING DISORDER: *Recovery for Adults with the Plate-by-Plate Approach®*
Copyright © 2023 by Wendy Sterling and Casey Crosbie
Insert photographs copyright © 2023 by The Experiment, LLC
Illustration on page 162 copyright © 2023 by Eva Musby, anorexiafamily.com
Exercise chart on page 182 reprinted with permission from Kate Bennett, PsyD (2023)

The Experiment, LLC | 220 East 23rd Street, Suite 600, New York, NY 10010-4658 | theexperimentpublishing.com

This book contains the opinions and ideas of its authors. It is intended to provide helpful and informative material on the subjects addressed in the book. It is sold with the understanding that the authors and publisher are not engaged in rendering medical, health, or any other kind of personal professional services in the book. The authors and publisher specifically disclaim all responsibility for any liability, loss, or risk—personal or otherwise—that is incurred as a consequence, directly or indirectly, of the use and application of any of the contents of this book.

THE PLATE-BY-PLATE APPROACH is a registered trademark of Wendy Sterling and Casey Crosbie.

THE EXPERIMENT and its colophon are registered trademarks of The Experiment, LLC. Many of the designations used by manufacturers and sellers to distinguish their products are claimed as trademarks. Where those designations appear in this book and The Experiment was aware of a trademark claim, the designations have been capitalized.

The Experiment's books are available at special discounts when purchased in bulk for premiums and sales promotions as well as for fundraising or educational use. For details, contact us at info@theexperimentpublishing.com.

Library of Congress Cataloging-in-Publication Data

Names: Sterling, Wendy, author. | Crosbie, Casey, author.
Title: How to nourish yourself through an eating disorder : recovery for
   adults with the plate-by-plate approach /
Wendy Sterling, MS, RD, CEDS-S, CSSD, Casey Crosbie, RD, CEDS-S.
Description: New York : The Experiment, 2023. | Includes bibliographical
   references and index.
Identifiers: LCCN 2023034814 (print) | LCCN 2023034815 (ebook) | ISBN
   9781615199778 | ISBN 9781615199785 (ebook)
Subjects: LCSH: Eating disorders--Diet therapy. | Eating disorders--Popular
   works. | Eating disorders--Treatment--Popular works.
Classification: LCC RC552.E18 S744 2023 (print) | LCC RC552.E18 (ebook) |
   DDC 616.85/26--dc23/eng/20230907
LC record available at https://lccn.loc.gov/2023034814
LC ebook record available at https://lccn.loc.gov/2023034815

ISBN 978-1-61519-977-8
Ebook ISBN 978-1-61519-978-5

Text and cover design, and insert photographs, by Beth Bugler
Photographs on pp. 53, 60, 85, 87, 88, 90, 91, 93, 94, 241 courtesy of the authors

Manufactured in the United States of America

First printing October 2023
10 9 8 7 6 5 4 3 2 1

DISCLAIMER

Please note, this book is for educational purposes only and is not a substitute for comprehensive eating disorder care.

PRIVILEGES

As two cis, White, heterosexual, thin, able-bodied women with financial security, we recognize that our bodies and unearned privileges do not necessarily represent that of our readers and may alter our perspective. We bring this book to you through our secondhand experience, as providers whose patients have "lived experience."

A NOTE ABOUT CASE EXAMPLES

Throughout this book we refer to case examples taken directly from our work with our patients over the years. All names have been changed to protect their privacy.

CONTENTS

Introduction: Why This Approach?   1

PART 1: Where to Begin

Chapter 1: Understanding Your Eating Disorder
and the Obsession with Food   8

Chapter 2: Signs and Symptoms of an Eating Disorder:
What Should I Look For?   19

PART 2: The Plate-by-Plate Approach®

Chapter 3: Conducting Your Baseline Nutrition Assessment   38

Chapter 4: Achieving the Plate   46

Chapter 5: Why This Plate Breakdown?   61

Chapter 6: Accelerated Nutritional Rehabilitation   77

Chapter 7: Putting It All Together: Meal and Snack Ideas   85

Chapter 8: An Approach for All   95

Chapter 9: Barriers to Following the Plate-by-Plate Approach® 108

PART 3: Common Issues and Strategies for Recovery

Chapter 10: Getting Help from Experts and Loved Ones   124

Chapter 11: Common Medical Issues (Lesley Williams, MD)   134

Chapter 12: Exploring Therapeutic Strategies for Recovery (Nan Shaw, LCSW, FBT, CEDS-S)   153

Chapter 13: To Exercise or Not: Managing Exercise and Dysfunctional Movement   173

Chapter 14: Pregnancy, Postpartum, and Parenting   190

PART 4: Food Freedom

Chapter 15: Moving Beyond Food Fears   212

Chapter 16: Four Steps to Freeing Yourself from Food Fears   224

Chapter 17: Navigating Real Life   236

Chapter 18: Increasing Body Satisfaction   250

Chapter 19: "I need you to know THIS!" (For Family and Friends in My Life)   261

Chapter 20: Normal Eating   271

Notes   283

Resources   303

Acknowledgments   307

Index   311

About the Authors and Contributors   328

INTRODUCTION:
WHY THIS APPROACH?

SEVENTY MILLION PEOPLE suffer from eating disorders (EDs) world-wide.[1] In the United States alone, twenty million women and ten million men suffer from a clinically significant ED at some point in their life. The most common EDs are anorexia nervosa, bulimia nervosa, binge eating disorder, or other specified feeding/eating disorder. Eating disorders can be life-threatening and if left untreated carry the second-highest mortality rate after opioid addiction.[2] EDs are associated with psychological impairment, significant comorbidities, medical complications, nutrient deficiencies, and suicidality.[3]

We have written this book as a tool for those suffering in silence, for those who have been misdiagnosed, ignored, shamed, scared to come forward, or who have unsuccessfully tried other treatments. Throughout this book you will hear that EDs don't discriminate, and they present in many different forms. We hope this book will help you not only meet your medical and nutritional needs for ED recovery but also reestablish a healthy relationship with food and your body.

EDs can affect anyone—of all sizes, genders, races, ethnicities, and age groups. No, you don't have to be "emaciated" to have an ED. In fact, you might be surprised to learn that less than 6 percent of those diagnosed with an ED are considered clinically "underweight."[4] You can't tell just by looking at someone whether they are sick or the *degree to which they are sick*. Yet many think, "I can't possibly be sick enough to warrant treatment." Or worse, the clinician they see misses it altogether.

Throughout, we will closely examine the signs and symptoms of EDs; the resultant medical complications; how therapy can help; physical and emotional effects in the presence of energy deficiency (RED-S); when to stop exercising; how to navigate pregnancy or menopause, how to achieve body acceptance, and of course, how adults can renourish themselves using the Plate-by-Plate Approach®.

We previously published *How to Nourish Your Child Through an Eating Disorder* for parents using a family-based treatment approach to support their child in recovery. Our first book introduced the Plate-by-Plate Approach®, a no-numbers, no-counting approach for nutritional rehabilitation using just a 10-inch dinner plate as the backbone. The approach asked parents to fill their child's plate with all 5 food groups, and to challenge the ED. Inherent in the philosophy is the importance of variety, with an emphasis on plating "what looks normal" rather than plating a certain number of calories—eventually allowing for a seamless transition to normal eating. In *How to Nourish Yourself Through an Eating Disorder*, we focus on adults, applying the same key principles to help with your recovery goals and to reestablish your relationship with food. Here, we have included tips that we use directly with our own adult patients that may be helpful to you while doing this work. This includes strategies for navigating the obstacles to one's recovery, including managing constipation, nausea, bloating, and sickness, or how to transition back to work, school, or travel during the recovery process.

The Plate-by-Plate Approach® can be applied across all diagnoses (see chapter 8). Each person's plan will look slightly different depending on their unique needs, based on age, biological sex, activity level, body size, and recovery goals. We'll walk you through the early stages of initiating a new meal plan and then adjusting it (if needed), and eventually preparing for the transition to normal eating.

You'll learn how to be successful not only at home but also while away, which is fundamental in recovery. In chapter 15, we will lead you through the process of being your own detective to assess your food fears and food rules. We will then discuss the process of "exposure," which encourages you, when ready, to experience some of the foods that escalate your anxiety.

Repeated experiences with these foods help to decrease anxiety. Being able to consume a variety of foods without fear is your ticket to normal eating, food freedom, and ultimately a lasting recovery.

Much has been written on what constitutes "recovery" from an ED, and for the most part, we follow the general belief that recovery is normalized eating, weight restoration for those who need it, resumption of menses or the normalization of hormones, improved overall health, as well as clearer thinking and actions. But recovery includes the many smaller victories that only those familiar with EDs will recognize—the ability to eat out at a restaurant with ease and even joy, the birthday cake received with happiness instead of dread, a successful trip, and a relative's random comment about your appearance that is simply ignored.

Our approach to nutrition is different from the ones usually employed, such as food measuring, calorie counting, and dividing food into "exchanges." EDs love numbers, counting, and measuring. Yet, counting calories, or counting macros, can be obsessive. Patients will count in their heads, on napkins, on their phones, on their hands . . . and many will say they don't like tracking their food this way but feel compelled to do so. "I feel like a virus has taken over my mind, and I need to be powered down. My mind is exploding with thoughts around food," one patient shared. A number of studies have shown that tracking apps cause psychological distress and ED symptoms.[5]

One of the most commonly used systems in ED treatment centers is the "exchange system," which is unlike what you'll find in this book. With the exchange system, an individual with an ED may be assigned a number of calories and an allotment of servings per food group that they can then "spend" as they wish. The exchanges allow for all foods to fit into a person's meal plan. However, there are many limitations. Restaurants, homemade foods, and recipes can be difficult to figure out. And some foods might have several exchanges attached to them, making the system feel complicated (example: lasagna might be 2 starch exchanges, 2 protein exchanges, 1 vegetable exchange, and 1 fat exchange). The exchanges can often be manipulated, too, with many people reporting that they choose the lowest-calorie items in each category, which throws off their daily caloric intake. The exchange system requires counting, measuring, and tallying throughout the day, which can increase obsessiveness around food and hold a person back from eating food that doesn't fit perfectly into their checklist. The exchange system was never meant to be for those in the later stages of recovery; instead people are eventually transitioned to intuitive eating. Yet, even when the exchange system is no longer part of their meal plans, many describe that when they look at their plates, remnants of the exchange system are floating around in their minds.

In 2011, the US Department of Agriculture (USDA) began to use a visual plate-model approach—MyPlate—to educate the general public about nutrition. They moved away from counting servings and moved toward creating "healthy messages" with a visual infographic of how much of each food group we should be eating. MyPlate replaced the food pyramid model. Our Plate-by-Plate Approach® is similar to the USDA's MyPlate in that it provides you with a visual representation of different food groups. However, MyPlate was created to combat the "obesity" epidemic with inherent messaging to "eat less" and "lose weight" (Note: Terms like "overweight" and "obesity" are considered to be stigmatizing, since they are separating people by weight; as such, we put these terms in quotes throughout the book). This messaging is the opposite of ED recovery; weight loss and dieting perpetuate EDs. Therefore, a plating system built on this premise is harmful to those with, or at risk for developing, an ED.

The Plate-by-Plate Approach® is a blank slate that does not involve counting, numbers, or measuring. Where the ED pulls for complexity, this approach strives for simplicity. You can choose from one of two plates (50% grains, 25% vegetables/fruits, 25% protein, with added dairy/dairy alternative and fats or 33% grains, 33% proteins, 33% fruits/vegetables, with added dairy/dairy alternative and fats), which can be further customized by adjusting the frequency and volume of snacks, depending on your nutritional needs.

Our approach considers the benefit of people never having to think of numbers, tracking, or counting, and the plate being just the plate from beginning to end, right down to recovery. Instead, the focus is on balance, variety, and what looks "normal." This tool can be used across many cultures and customized by dietary needs. We ask people we work with what foods they eat in their household, their culture. We use their answers to support their recovery. Unlike "diets," the ideas presented as part of this approach are not mandates. Fundamental to this approach is that there is flexibility, just as in normal eating. This helps to reduce the shame that might go along with having "a meal plan" or needing to follow certain restrictions. Having flexibility allows for our patients to feel more seen and heard.

In some cultures, vegetables are not separated, so the plate might look different from what we are explaining here—and that's perfectly acceptable and welcomed. Some of our patients with limited preferences won't eat a vegetable, or some will eat only fruit. There is so much customization possible within this approach. It can be followed exactly or loosely. Most important is that this approach provides the structure to think about volume of food, snacks, regularity, variety, and consistency. Take aspects that work for you and leave others behind.

Plating food at once, on a 10-inch plate, may not align with certain cultural practices and styles of eating. Cultures in which there is an emphasis on eating from bowls (as seen in many Asian cultures), using hands to eat off shared dishes (common in certain African cultures), or eating small meals throughout the day may not benefit from this approach. Trying to follow along with an approach that utilizes plates when that style of eating is not natural for someone might add even more confusion around food. That said, we do discuss how to use this approach when plating soups like ramen and pho, and we aim to make this approach as culturally broad and useful as possible.

We are eager to share more about the Plate-by-Plate Approach® and how it can be used for adults with EDs, and we hope we have delivered this information in as inclusive a way as possible. We use it for most clients in our practice, and now we share it with you. We hope this book provides what you need to renourish yourself through your ED and to reestablish a healthy relationship with food.

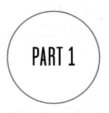

PART 1

Where to Begin

CHAPTER 1

Understanding Your Eating Disorder and the Obsession with Food

EATING BEHAVIORS THAT feel off deserve help. A few examples of behaviors that can interfere with your sense of peace around mealtime include vomiting after meals, skipping meals, bingeing, restricting calories, excessively exercising, hoarding food, counting calories, saving calories, feeling stressed at mealtime, and chewing and spitting.

While EDs appear to be focused around food and weight, dieting, or "clean eating" on a deeper level, EDs are complex brain disorders that often serve as a sophisticated coping mechanism for stressful or overwhelming emotions or situations. EDs are not about vanity or a lack of control. Those who are diagnosed with an ED may have a combination of factors that create the perfect storm for these illnesses to develop. This includes a person's individual traits such as genetics and psychological makeup; aggravating factors such as depression, anxiety, or OCD; or personal life experiences, including trauma, a history of being bullied, and more. These are often combined with social factors, such as divorce, death of a loved one, poor living conditions, and cultural and external social pressure, including the influence of peers. Additionally, co-occurring medical diagnoses (such as irritable bowel syndrome, celiac disease, diabetes mellitus) that place restrictions on one's diet can cause an increased risk for the development of an ED.[1]

Dieting

Body image dissatisfaction is common, develops early, and stems in part from a weight-obsessed society and dieting culture that constantly tells you that "your body is wrong." An emphasis on weight loss and a "thin ideal" can lead to the development of body dissatisfaction and EDs.[2] In fact, an eight-year study by Stice and colleagues found that the "perceived pressure to be thin" was a primary risk factor for developing an ED.[3] Poor body image can start very early in life. A study looking at body image development showed that even by age six, young girls are already preoccupied with their weight and shape.[4]

Diets don't actually work. A study of nearly seventeen thousand children, ages nine to fourteen, found that dieting was a significant predictor of weight gain and led to increased rates of binge eating in both girls and boys.[5] Additional studies show that the more a person diets, the more weight they gain over time.[6] Weight teasing by peers and family members (occurring in 37 percent larger-bodied girls, and 40 percent larger-bodied boys) predicts weight gain, binge eating, and extreme weight control measures.[7] Dieting is the biggest predictor of EDs. A 2016 report by the American Academy of Pediatrics (AAP) concluded that dieting is "counterproductive" and increases the risk of developing an ED.[8] It is therefore not surprising to see high rates of disordered eating and dieting throughout the life span.

Eating Disorders in Adulthood

EDs can occur at any age and can develop for the first time during midlife or reemerge in midlife after a long period of recovery in previous years or decades. And of course, in some, EDs are chronic and continue throughout life. According to Margo Maine, in her interview with Kathy Cortese on the *ED Matters* podcast, "Eating disorders are more prevalent than breast cancer in women over fifty."[9] This is an astounding statistic, considering that breast cancer is the second most common cancer in women in the US (the first is skin cancer). One in eight American women will develop invasive breast cancer over the course of their lifetime.[10] Triggers for EDs that occur late in life include menopause and hormone changes, empty nest syndrome, divorce, retirement, death of a loved one, declining health and mobility, increased stressors, isolation, and body changes.

Anorexia nervosa is the most common ED among people over fifty, with women affected most often, and is associated with other psychiatric disorders and overall shorter life span.[11] Shape and weight concerns have been shown to peak for males around aged fifty-five to sixty-four.[12] Overall, inpatient medical hospitalizations for women over 35 increase over time.[13]

There are barriers for older people getting into treatment. There can be an increase in shame with the thought, "I am too old to have an eating disorder." Responsibilities such as work, running the house, or taking care of kids or grandkids might get in the way of treatment. Or, there might be other barriers, such as needing to take care of sick family members, financial constraints, or treatment interfering with retirement plans. For those who have had the ED for decades, some may falsely think it's "not as bad" as when they were younger.

"The scaffolding of the ED may have been with them, perhaps for decades. It is terrifying to think of losing this thing that has helped them and, in many instances, defined them. And families around them often think, 'Well that's just who Mom is . . . that's just who my sibling is,'" shares Ibbits Newhall, Eating Disorder Treatment Resource Consultant, cocreator of the Recovery Roadmap Series for Families. And then, should an older adult finally make their way into treatment, there can be a sense of "otherness" if the program doesn't specially cater to older people. Working through these barriers is important, as treatment delays worsen the severity of symptoms.

Another at-risk stage of life is during pregnancy, when a person experiences great physical and emotional changes. Preconception nutrition is critical to conceiving as well as to the development of a healthy baby. Adequate nutrition throughout pregnancy, as well as reaching weight milestones, ensures the placenta is able to grow and nourish the developing baby. Nausea, heartburn, constipation, gas, and/or medical concerns such as anemia and gestational diabetes make pregnancy a highly risky time requiring close medical, nutritional, and psychological monitoring for those with EDs.

Eating Disorder Diagnoses

An ED is diagnosed by health professionals using diagnostic criteria from the *Diagnostic and Statistical Manual of Mental Disorders, Fifth Edition* (DSM-5). The DSM-5 lists the following eating/feeding disorders: anorexia nervosa (AN), bulimia nervosa (BN), avoidant/restrictive food intake disorder (ARFID), other specified feeding or eating disorder (OSFED), binge eating disorder (BED), pica, and rumination disorder.[14]

Anorexia nervosa was previously diagnosed when someone reached a very low weight, lost their menstrual cycle, had a distorted body image, and was fearful of gaining weight. The most recent definition of anorexia nervosa published in the DSM-5 has removed the low weight criteria, and the diagnosis can be made without regard to menstrual status. The newer diagnostic criteria are more inclusive, capturing those who are suffering regardless of weight and menstrual status.

"Atypical anorexia" (AAN) is technically a subcategory of OSFED and is used to describe those who meet all the same criteria as AN but the individual's weight remains within or above the "normal" range. Like AN, patients with AAN may have lost a significant amount of body weight, be severely malnourished, and medically and psychiatrically unstable. Weight gain will be necessary for renourishment, to improve metabolic functioning, hormones, and vital signs.

The use of the word "atypical" by the medical community is stigmatizing, as it differentiates patients by weight—yet, all patients with AN and AAN are struggling with the same psychological and medical complications. Atypical AN is quite possibly more typical than AN; patients with AAN make up about 50 percent of the patients admitted to medical hospital units, and 34 percent of outpatient settings.[15] Patients with AAN might be living in larger bodies, where weight loss may be praised and celebrated by family members and health providers. This can cause these patients to experience a ten- or eleven-month delay in getting treatment, often due to provider weight bias,[16] with providers missing the chance to make an earlier diagnosis.

The criterion for bulimia nervosa was adjusted in the DSM-5 from bingeing and purging three times per week for three months, to bingeing once per week for three months. A binge is defined as eating, in a discrete period of time (e.g., within any two-hour period), an amount of food that is definitely larger than most people would eat during a similar period of time, and a sense of lack of control while eating during the episode (e.g., a feeling that one cannot stop eating or control what or how much one is eating). In bulimia nervosa, there is a "compensatory" mechanism present, such as vomiting, laxative use, diuretics, exercise, or even restricting.

BED (binge-eating disorder) is is more than three times more common than AN and BN, and approximately 40 percent of those with BED are male.[17] Unlike bulimia nervosa, BED is not associated with a compensatory mechanism. Binge eating occurs, on average, at least once a week for three months. Here, the diagnosis of bingeing is expanding to include three or more of the following.

1. Eating much more rapidly than normal

2. Eating until feeling uncomfortably full

3. Eating large amounts of food when not feeling physically hungry

4. Eating alone because of feeling embarrassed by how much one is eating

5. Feeling disgusted with oneself, depressed, or very guilty afterward

6. Feeling marked distress regarding binge eating is present

Those with EDs don't always fit into one diagnostic box; many exhibit characteristics across several different eating-disorder diagnoses. The diagnosis "other specified feeding or eating disorder" (OSFED) refers to those who have significant distress around food and weight but who do not meet the full criteria for any of the other EDs. For example, our client Julia was struggling with bingeing at night but not with the frequency that is defined to meet the criteria in BED. Therefore, she would likely fall into a diagnosis of OSFED for now, but this could change. There is likely a high prevalence of those with OSFED, since it captures behaviors from many types EDs and captures many aspects of disordered eating.

Disordered eating can fall across a spectrum in which one may fluctuate from being symptom-free to disordered eating, all the way through a diagnosed clinical ED. Some may find that their ED moves back and forth along the spectrum based on their life experiences, mood, stress, financial status, and other factors. Similarly, the EDs of athletes can vary based on training cycle, season, pressure, health status, or with playing time.[18]

Spectrum of Eating Behavior[19]

Optimized nutrition: Safe, supported, purposeful, and individualized nutrition practices that best balance health and performance

Disordered eating: Problematic eating behavior that fails to meet the clinical diagnosis for an eating disorder

Eating disorder: Behavior that meets DSM-5 diagnostic criteria for a feeding and eating disorder

Muscle dysmorphia, a subtype of body dysmorphic disorder as per the DSM-5 diagnostic criteria, has been commonly referred to as "bigorexia" or "reverse anorexia."[20] Here there is a preoccupation with being muscular and constant worry that one is not sufficiently muscular. There is a distortion, such that a person's muscle mass is actually considered normal or even objectively muscular. The quest for muscularity is all-consuming and obsessive. It dominates one's thoughts and actions, with the person spending hours in the gym and excessive amounts of money on supplements and vitamins. This intense preoccupation is associated with depression and anxiety.[21] The person might exhibit some of these characteristics, though no official criteria have been established.[22]

1. They might engage in muscle enhancing behaviors, which include extreme dieting, anabolic steroid use (higher in this group), excessive exercise, and protein supplement consumption. This should be differentiated from those using the supplements to improve sports performance.

2. There might be an intentional covering up of the body—an avoidance of tight clothing, instead opting for baggy sweats (even during the summer). Body checking is common. A person may show certain parts of their body only after doing bicep curls or push-ups to "make the muscles look bigger."

3. A person might feel extreme anxiety, embarrassment, or an avoidance of revealing one's physique while changing clothes.

4. They may have aesthetic versus sports-performance-related goals. Goals will be confined to building muscle ("size, definition, leanness") particularly in the chest, biceps, and abdomen, with a focus on how the body looks versus how the body performs.

5. There is a prioritization of weight training and workouts above all else, above one's social life, work, and personal life.

6. There will be trouble taking a rest day, tapering, or with periodizing (adjusting one's training intensity according to the season or around an event).

The diagnosis of avoidant/restrictive food intake disorder typically does not have weight or body-image concerns, but these individuals have trouble meeting their energy needs and may have unintentionally lost a significant amount of weight. They may have sensitivities to texture, taste, smell, and temperatures, or they may fear an aversive consequence such as pain, choking, vomiting, nausea, trouble swallowing, or an allergic reaction. There can be a suppressed appetite due to stress and anxiety. Some may describe a lifelong lack of interest in food, and a persistent low appetite, which make day-to-day feeding challenging.

There might be a history of feeding difficulties, intolerances, or allergies that may contribute to early aversive experiences with eating. An overlay of medical or gastrointestinal complications may exist, such as eosinophilic esophagitis, celiac disease, or inflammatory bowel syndrome, making feeding more complicated.[23] Additionally, autism spectrum disorder (ASD) and attention deficit hyperactivity disorder (ADHD) appear to be more frequent in individuals with ARFID.[24]

Those with ARFID may have limited preferences, and specific food requests from certain places. For example, they may enjoy eating a burger, but from only one restaurant and not from others, or they may request food prepared in specific ways. They may never have tried certain fruits and vegetables and may love desserts and chips.

Eating Disorders in Men

EDs have historically been thought to be something that affected mostly women. However, there has been an increasing prevalence of men being diagnosed with EDs, too, which has been rising at a faster rate than women.[25] Men face pressure to be lean and muscular and are bombarded with images of six-pack abs and chiseled biceps. There tends to be a focus among men, which is not typically seen among women, on getting bigger. To gain weight, men turn to such muscle-enhancing behaviors as increasing protein intake or taking creatine or other supplements while cutting calories to increase leanness. There can be an emphasis on fasting, purging, or using laxatives. There is so little education about what an ED looks like in a man that it is unfortunately far too common for a health provider to miss making an ED diagnosis. Often, the person may not even realize their behaviors are concerning, blending in with gym culture, the environment of athletics, and how "guys eat," making it hard to see that these behaviors are concerning and should be mentioned to a professional.

Andrew Walen, LCSW-C, LICSW, CEDS-S, founder of D.U.D.E Mental Health and author of *Man Up to Eating Disorders*, describes his own ED as follows.

My behaviors look like typical male behaviors. I was a gym rat, never satisfied with my effort unless I hit personal bests. I was hyper-focused on performance metrics. I hated my binges, which were common as I starved myself during the day, so they were typically in secret at home with large take-out or drive-through meals. When I did eat out it was often at places like Indian buffets with other guy friends, where my binges looked like typical male behavior. Seeing who could stack up more empty plates was almost competitive and fun and seen as masculine.

EDs thrive in secrecy, and many people avoid treatment or feel shame or embarrassment about having an ED, which has been (mistakenly) perceived as a "teen girl's problem."[26] This can be isolating and inevitably causes a delay in treatment, allowing the ED symptoms to escalate and exist for a longer period of time. A 2016 study found that when men were finally assessed by medical providers specializing in the treatment of EDs, many were orthostatic and bradycardic, and over 50 percent met criteria for inpatient hospitalization.[27] "Guys need help!" says Andrew Walen. "And they are coming in ever greater numbers to treatment. But there are few resources, little research for evidence-based practice, and almost no training provided to help these clients and that needs to change."

Men make up less than 1 percent of the ED research, and there remain many gaps in the treatment recommendations as a result. Should men seek treatment, programs are 90 percent female, leading men to feel more isolated and alone.

Additionally, the research studying best practices and treatment options is largely done on white subjects and through a white lens. More research, understanding, and education are needed to understand how men experience EDs.

Eating Disorders in BIPOC Communities

There has been an escalation of EDs among the BIPOC (Black, indigenous, people of color) community. Data from England's publicly funded National Health Service showed that hospital admissions for EDs are rising faster in minority populations than in white ones.[28]

The rise in EDs in the BIPOC community is in part due to failure of clinicians to recognize EDs in marginalized communities.[29] People who are BIPOC are asked about ED symptoms significantly less than those who are white.[30] Certain cultural values or expectations around strength or privacy, stigma around mental health concerns, and pressure around food and body might also cause someone to be less likely to come forward about their disorder. There can also be a lack of education, difficulty in accessing health care, and inequities in health care. This delay in recognizing there is an issue and accessing treatment can make the ED harder to treat, eventually requiring greater intervention.

"Because of the historic context of how the medical and psychological community has mistreated Black Americans there has, over time, developed medical mistrust within the community," explains Kyra Ross, MsED, MHC-LP, a psychotherapist, in an article for Verywell Mind. "In addition to the experienced medical mistrust, there is currently an enormous discrepancy in access to quality health care between white Americans and Black Americans," she adds. Additional barriers to treatment for treating EDs in the Black community include a lack of education, difficult relationships with food, and treatment inequities.[31]

Another important barrier for treatment experienced by the BIPOC community is the lack of diversity and bias among ED providers. When a person enters a treatment center, the centers themselves can reinforce a sense of "otherness" to BIPOC clients, our patients have shared with us. This can be reinforced by a lack of diversity among providers, and again, if the program doesn't support your cultural meal practices.

Eating Disorders in LGBTQ+ Communities

EDs and disordered eating are more common among LGBT adults and adolescents than among those who are heterosexual and cisgender.[32] Those with gender dysphoria might use the ED to suppress secondary sex characteristics, hormones, menstruation, breast development, or unwanted changes their body. Transgender individuals have higher rates of disordered eating and body image dissatisfaction than cisgendered people.[33] There is also higher risk of developing an ED for those who identify as two spirit, lesbian, gay, bisexual, transgender, queer/questioning, intersex, asexual (2SLGBTQIA+).[34] BIPOC 2SLGBTQIA+ face layered stigma. There are few studies examining ED pathology in gender-nonbinary people. In one study, nonbinary adults had three times greater odds of AN and BN compared to transgender men or women.[35]

LGBTQ individuals are more likely to face discrimination, social stigma, oppression, and to lack social support, all heightening risk factors for an ED. "Queer folks receive messages on a daily basis that their bodies and core identities are unacceptable, unimportant, or at worst, repulsive," says Equip therapist Carise Rotach. "Layer these messages with eating disorder thoughts—both internal and externally confirmed by society—and it can often feel like they are swimming upstream."[36]

Stereotypes about EDs existing in "straight, white, affluent girls," an acronym known as "SWAG," leads to overlooking underrecognized populations. The diagnosis is often missed among males, those living in larger bodies, in BIPOC and other minority groups, in older individuals, and among those from poorer communities.

CHAPTER 2

Signs and Symptoms of an Eating Disorder: What Should I Look For?

SEVERAL COMMON CHARACTERISTICS in various categories are typically seen in EDs: physical signs, behaviors around food and exercise, body image, and cognitive/mood changes. Having done this work for decades, we are still seeing new behaviors each day. If you are experiencing any of the signs or symptoms mentioned in this chapter, we suggest checking in with a health professional (medical doctor, therapist, or dietitian) as soon as possible. These behaviors do not have to be dramatic or terrifying in order for you to justify seeking help. Symptoms might appear quietly, like gentle knocks, which are signs that your body and mind need help. Don't ignore them. They are unlikely to get better on their own, and the prognosis for fighting EDs is much better when caught early.[1]

In the next few pages, we present a list of characteristics and behaviors that are commonly seen with EDs. Some people may experience only a few of these symptoms, whereas others will experience many.

Signs of an Eating Disorder

CHANGES IN FOOD BEHAVIORS	PHYSICAL SIGNS
Increased interest in food and exercise	Weight changes (loss or gain)
Dieting	Cessation of period (unrelated to menopause)
Bingeing	Decreased sex drive
Increased rigidity, rules, and lack of flexibility	Dry skin, dry hair, brittle nails
Sorting foods into good foods and bad foods	Frequent injuries
Taking health messages to the extreme	Frequent stress fractures
Lack of spontaneity	Dizziness
Lack of variety	Hair loss /thinner hair
Plain, dry food	Orange hands/feet (hypercarotenemia)
Unable to eat outside the home	Always feeling cold (hypothermia)
Compensatory behaviors	Fine hair on face (lanugo)
Abnormal food behaviors	Bloating
Unusual food combinations	Heart racing
Eating slowly	
Dissecting food and messy eating	
Orthorexia: focus on "clean eating"	

EXERCISE	BODY IMAGE
Excess movement	Increased focus on body weight and shape
Shaking	Body checking
Standing	Body image distress
Longer-than-usual workouts or training	

COGNITIVE AND PSYCHOLOGICAL CHANGES
Brain fog
Social withdrawal
Increased anxiety/depression
Irritability
Decreased concentration

Changes in Food Behaviors

Increased interest in food and exercise

You might find you are more interested in health and wellness. Perhaps you saw something on Instagram or received lab work from your medical doctor, who recommended you make a change. Nothing's wrong with cooking more or becoming interested in nutrition unless it starts to take over your life, limit your functioning, and/or becomes an obsession.

Dieting

Dieting often looks and feels like an ED and is not compatible with recovery. We see behaviors such as counting calories, tracking food in apps, weighing and measuring food, weighing and measuring yourself, and recording these measurements. This often comes with an interest in food, cooking, recipes, and watching cooking shows.

Bingeing

Bingeing is a hallmark criterion for BED. The clinical definition of a binge is eating larger amounts of food over a period of time and feeling out of control (see page 12 for more on the definition of binge eating). Additional characteristics such as eating rapidly, eating beyond fullness, eating when not hungry, feeling embarrassed/ashamed/disgusted by bingeing, and more, are outlined earlier in this book.

Increased rigidity, rules, and lack of flexibility

EDs love rules, such as, "I won't eat after seven PM." or "I will not have a midday dessert." Some people will have ritualistic eating practices, requiring meals to occur in a certain order, at a certain time, or with certain foods consumed first. Foods might not be allowed to touch each other on the plate. Or one's favorite food items might be consumed last. Those with strict guidelines around food, including how food should be prepared, find it challenging to navigate restaurants, family meals, barbecues, concerts, parties, or traveling. We discuss increasing flexibility and food freedom in chapter 16.

Sorting foods into good and bad

Often, we see people categorizing foods as "good" and "bad." "Good foods" are typically foods a person considers to be "healthy." Examples of good foods include fruit, yogurt, vegetables, chicken breast, and fish. Conversely, bad foods, also known as "fear foods," are foods that feel scary to eat. A person may label a food as "fattening," "disgusting," "unhealthy," "gross," or "too high in sugar." Fear foods might include potato chips, hamburgers, ice cream, pizza, cookies, soda, and candy. This polarization of foods disconnects us from our body's wisdom and perpetuates a false belief that one food by itself has the power to alter health or weight. Persisting in this belief generates a high level of anxiety around food, preventing a person from achieving food freedom.

Taking health messages to the extreme

The rise in heart disease, diabetes, and cancer have caused society to focus on diet and exercise.[2] Exaggerated, extreme responses to nutrition information are common. If drinking water is good for you, drinking water all day must be better! That misguided thinking can be dangerous. The media have gone after juice, red meat, sugar, and white flour, and many people we work with have stopped eating these foods—*ever again for eternity*—despite these messages not being meant for them, or meant to be implemented in moderation. For instance, the Cleveland Clinic has recommended eating red meat several times a week (with smaller portions if there is history of high cholesterol).[3]

Lack of spontaneity

EDs don't like spontaneity. Here are some questions to consider.

- If your friends are going out for dinner, can you join them?
- If they're going out at an odd time when you normally wouldn't expect to eat, can you join in anyway?
- Does it bother you to take an extra bite of food outside of your set meals and snacks? For example, can you sample food at a farmers market or taste someone's homemade sauce or baked good?

The ability to have a random bite of food, out of turn without anxiety, is part of "normal" eating. Being spontaneous and carefree with food might look like grabbing a handful of chips between meals or taking a bite of a friend's meal. Or it might mean not feeling stressed and anxious around food. As someone becomes more obsessed with dieting, their food spontaneity may vanish. They may be counting calories in their head or feel like they need to manage or control their food as much as possible. Those who are following a meal plan may be fearful of eating other than what they believe they *should* eat. The ability to be spontaneous is a gateway to freedom from rigidity around food. Spontaneity tends to return over time as a person approaches true recovery.

Lack of variety

There may be little to no variety in food choices at meals and snacks, not only throughout the day but also throughout the week. We will take a closer look at variety in your meals and snacks when we explore your seven-day food record in chapter 3. Limited consumption of food within each food group might intensify one's fear of food and limit the ability to get as many nutrients as possible.

Plain, dry food

Some people eat a very plain diet without any sauce or flavor. Foods may be steamed, microwaved, and roasted without any oil. There may be an avoidance of fats, processed foods, cooked foods, and a desire to have foods in their most "natural form." Those with EDs may feel sauces are unhealthy and should be avoided. Some eat salad without dressing. Fats add flavor and texture and help to absorb nutrients. The combination of spices and flavors brings out the tastes of different ingredients in the dish. Eating is all about what feels good to you, and no one can argue with your preferences. But ask yourself if this is what *you* like, or what *your ED* demands?

Unable to eat outside the home

As the ED becomes more restrictive, so does what and where you eat. While you might have previously enjoyed going to lunch with friends or grabbing dinner with colleagues, now you might find that you are scared to have to "deal with the food." The anxiety might be so high that it feels easier to just eat at home. We explore how to expand your preferences, including to restaurants, in chapter 16.

Compensatory behaviors

A compensatory behavior, defined as a behavior used to eliminate the calories consumed, is a hallmark feature of BN and also present in AN and OSFED. Compensatory behaviors can include vomiting after meals; excessive exercise; misuse of laxatives, diuretics, diet pills, and teas; or a period of food restriction. Burning off calories, restricting food, or exercising after eating are all seen as forms of attempting to "get rid of" the calories consumed. These behaviors have dangerous medical complications, and will be explored further in chapter 11.

Abnormal eating behaviors and food combinations

Many eating behaviors have been observed among those struggling with their relationship to food. Mealtime behaviors noted among those with anorexia nervosa, and not seen in healthy controls, include staring at food, tearing food, nibbling or picking, dissecting food, excessive use of napkins to wipe grease or sauces off food or to hide food, inappropriate utensil use, hand fidgeting, and delaying eating.[4] We have also seen people who combine foods in an atypical way, such as oatmeal with ketchup. There might be an excessive use of salt, pepper, spices, soy sauce, balsamic vinegar, or hot sauce—spices and condiments that add flavor but don't add calories. Often in EDs, the body and mind are starved for calories and seek out a more intense flavor.[5]

We often find that assembling meals that are "cohesive" can be an issue for those with EDs. The items may be thrown together, some hot, some cold, and don't particularly complement each other. For example, a meal might be "bulgur, guacamole, a string cheese, and broccoli" or "one cup of miso soup, canned tuna, cereal, and blueberries." We also see people who use what might seem like the wrong utensil for the food being consumed. For example, someone might eat yogurt with a fork, allowing it to take longer to eat as it spills through. Or they might use a baby spoon instead of a regular spoon or chopsticks to eat cereal.

Eating slowly

Pacing can be an issue for many people, with meals taking hours to complete and with one meal leading into the next.

Dissecting food and messy eating

Ripping apart food, dissecting it, eating in a messy way, or letting food drop makes it very hard to ensure that all the food that you should be eating is actually eaten.

Table Behaviors

Below is a quick reference list for table behaviors to watch out for as you move forward in recovery. Most of these table behaviors are not allowed in ED treatment programs. Note: someone with special needs, a medical or neurological condition, or someone who has difficulty chewing or swallowing may not be able to adhere to some of the suggestions listed below. Careful consideration should be allowed for your unique needs before defaulting to blaming the ED. For example, someone with a dental device may have trouble eating cleanly; in that case, they might need a little extra food to make up for what was lost.

If there is a reason you can't adhere to a guideline on this list, skip over it. If you are working with a support team or in a program, please share those reasons with them. Perhaps you can recruit help from loved ones to work on normalizing whichever eating behaviors you feel need work, if any.

- Cutting food into tiny pieces
- Ripping and pulling apart foods
- Eating slowly or taking small bites
- Excessive fluid intake with meals or snacks

- Eating rapidly
- Organizing food on the plate before eating
- Eating foods in a specific order
- Letting food drop on the floor or table or spilling beverages
- Hiding food (under dishes or napkins)
- Spitting food into napkins
- Excessive use of napkins to wipe the mouth, hands, or silverware
- Constantly talking about food during the meal
- Shaking legs or moving excessively in any way
- Standing while eating

Throughout the process of returning to health, often known as "refeeding" or "nutritional rehabilitation," food choices improve and obsessions about food decrease in frequency and intensity.[6] The best chance for reducing obsessiveness and preoccupation with food is to achieve a balanced, healthy diet that meets your unique energy requirements.

Orthorexia: an intensified focus on health and dieting

An extreme version of "health consciousness" has been called "orthorexia." Not an official ED diagnosis, it does not appear in the DSM-5. Coined by Dr. Steven Bratman in his popular book *Health Food Junkies*, orthorexia refers to an all-encompassing obsession with health and nutrition and are preoccupied with "eating healthy" and "eating clean" to an excessively intrusive degree. Someone with orthorexia will likely exhibit many of the same behavioral signs seen in EDs, such as obsessive thinking and having a limited diet with rigid rules, but they may or may not have body image concerns seen in other EDs. They may also be at an appropriate weight, medically stable, and with normal hormone levels.

There tends to be a focus on quality over quantity and on achieving "perfect health" over losing weight. Those with orthorexia want each food selected to have "maximum nutritional benefit." They may choose foods that are free of additives, homemade, have minimal ingredients, are low-sugar, organic, cage-free, grass-fed, free-range, and high in fiber. They might feel superior to others, thinking they are eating better than everyone else, and may look down on the diet of others—at times even trying to educate or correct them. They may spend an inordinate amount of time in farmers markets, speaking directly to farmers to source their food. And in a wellness world of quinoa, cauliflower rice, and zoodles, it's easy to blend in.

With the influx of health messages, orthorexia has become increasingly common and can be debilitating. Many who are looking to "become healthy" are attracted to this messaging, yet an extreme adherence to these messages can, ironically, cause someone to become "unhealthy." As with traditional EDs, consequences of orthorexia include increased irritability, depression, anxiety, poor relationships with others, social avoidance, feelings of guilt, and an excessive amount of time spent thinking about or preparing meals, which takes time away from other activities.

Exercise

Dysfunctional movement

It's common to see changes in movement that correspond with one's ED. The intensity or duration of workouts might increase, or exercise might become dysfunctional. Dysfunctional movement exists when someone feels like they can't stop moving or feels compelled to move. The person believes that if they don't keep moving, there will be a negative consequence. There is often a high level of distress if unable to do their workout, and movement is prioritized above all other activities: family, social life, religious activities, and so on. Someone struggling with compulsive exercise may go up and down the stairs several extra times, contract their abdomen mid-conversation, walk the dog longer or more frequently, or run in place in the shower. A person might be exhausted or injured but train anyway. We will talk more about exercise and EDs in chapter 13, including what a balanced versus unbalanced relationship with movement looks like.

No movement

On the contrary, as one's EDs develops, we might see someone who was previously active stop being active. This change is often a red flag, as it can indicate a change in mood, energy balance, or body image.

Shaking, standing, fidgeting

Frequent standing, fidgeting, moving, and stair climbing is known as "NEAT," non-exercise activity thermogenesis. Movement, as measured by an accelerometer, was shown to be more prominent in those with anorexia nervosa compared to controls.[7]

Physical Signs

Weight changes (loss or gain)

Typically, weight loss or gain signifies a change in energy balance. Changes in weight could be a sign that you're eating less or more erratically, overexercising, avoiding exercising, bingeing, purging, using laxatives or diuretics, engaging in disordered eating behaviors, having fluid shifts, or having a troubled relationship with food. It is normal to have fluctuations in one's weight throughout life, as well as throughout the month due to hormonal fluctuations. Certain medications can cause weight fluctuations. It is also normal and expected for there to be weight gain as people age. However, large weight fluctuations that occur may often reflect inconsistencies in one's food intake, such as bingeing, restricting, or going for long periods of time without eating, or having signal gastrointestinal concerns like constipation, edema (water retention), and other medical concerns. These signs could be a red flag for something more serious happening.

Dizziness

It's not normal to feel dizzy when you get out of bed in the morning or when you get up from sitting after a long period of time. Dizziness can be a sign you are not eating or hydrating enough, and consequently you could have vital sign instabilities such as orthostasis (changes in pulse or blood pressure due to gravitational shifts when you stand up) or bradycardia (low heart rate). Certain medications and medical conditions can cause dizziness, and this is why we suggest consulting a doctor immediately if you feel dizzy. Note: Not everyone who is struggling with their relationship to food or exercise will feel dizzy, so don't mistake your lack of dizziness to mean that everything is fine.

Cessation of menstruation

In biological females, dieting, bingeing, chaotic eating, losing weight, skipping meals, purging, using laxatives, and/or overexercising are examples of how disordered eating can alter one's menstrual cycle. The stopping of one's menstrual cycle when unrelated to perimenopause or menopause is a physiological sign that the body is out of balance. This occurs when an individual has lost too much weight or when their caloric intake is insufficient.[8] If an energy imbalance exists, one's periods may become irregular (oligomenorrhea) or absent (amenorrhea; defined as the skipping of three menstrual cycles or more). Dieting alone can be enough to alter one's menstrual cycle, as the body lacks sufficient energy to support its systems and turns off nonessential functions like menstruation. While it's common for athletes to skip their menstrual periods, it is not normal. There are many reasons for an individual to have an abnormal menstrual cycle, and a workup by a medical provider can be helpful.

Decreased sex drive

Reduced food intake and/or weight loss can suppress hormones, such as estrogen and testosterone. For biological females, decreased hormones will result in menstrual cycles becoming either irregular, late, shorter, or missed entirely. Biological males can see a reduction in testosterone level and may notice fewer morning erections. Healthy males usually have several erections throughout the night as sleep cycles end, which corresponds to normal blood flow.[9] Testosterone levels may peak in the morning, which is why many biological males may see a morning erection, usually at the end of a sleep cycle.

Testosterone levels tend to be highest for young adults and throughout one's thirties and tend to decrease thereafter. However, during times of malnutrition, there can be a sudden decrease. A suppression in hormones can translate to decreased libido or decreased vaginal lubrication.

Dry skin, dry hair, brittle nails

Malnutrition can cause dry skin, dry hair, and brittle nails. While cold weather can have an effect on skin condition, we also know that the skin reflects how our body is doing on the inside. Our skin and hair need nutrients such as protein, zinc, vitamin C, biotin, calories, fats, and fluids to thrive.[10] If our body is not getting the nutrients it needs, we will see the result show up as dry, flaky skin, dry hair, and brittle nails. Nails need protein and calcium to harden.

Hair loss or thinning

Visible hair loss or thinning might not be noticeable until about three months after the peak of malnutrition. During malnutrition, the hair follicles go into a resting phase—there is not enough fuel to stimulate normal hair growth and regeneration. Hair loss can sometimes increase during refeeding, as the hair cycle wakes up and begins to produce new hair, causing hair that was stuck in the resting phase to fall out. This can be alarming for many people, especially if they have begun to eat more, but it signals that the body is getting back on track. Hair loss might last weeks or months but usually improves with time.

Frequent injuries

Insufficient food intake is associated with an increase in injuries. In fact, injuries among athletes with disordered eating are more common than among those with a balanced relationship with food.[11]

Frequent stress fractures

Low bone density is one of the most prominent complications of low estrogen (as seen with irregular or absent menses) and low testosterone levels.[12] The duration of amenorrhea (loss of period) caused by low estrogen levels, or the duration of low testosterone levels, is correlated to low bone mineral density, which is associated with osteoporosis and leads to a high fracture rate.

Orange hands/feet (hypercarotenemia)

Some people notice their hands and feet turn orange. Excessive intake of beta-carotene resulting from overconsumption of fruits and vegetables (think whole bags of baby carrots or several red peppers or plates of vegetables in one sitting) can cause the skin to take on a yellow or orange hue. This usually occurs in the context of an unbalanced diet (not enough fats, starches, proteins), not enough total calories, and often in the context of malnutrition. Beta-carotene is a pigment found in many fruits and vegetables, such as carrots, dark leafy greens, winter squash, sweet potatoes, and cantaloupe. Normally, the body converts beta-carotene to vitamin A, eliminating the presence of any abnormal pigment in the skin. Hypercarotenemia is especially pronounced on the palms of the hands, the soles of the feet, and, to a lesser degree, the face.

Always feeling cold

You may have also noticed that you always feel cold. This is known as "cold intolerance." Your hands and feet might feel cold, and you may be bundling up when others are wearing T-shirts. Sweatshirts and sweaters may also make it easier to hide your body. During malnutrition, it is common to see a bluish discoloration (acrocyanosis) to the tips of the fingers as well as on the nose and ears. The body lacks the energy to maintain cardiovascular function to keep your body warm and is prioritizing sending blood to the most vital organs. Bruising and skin sores are due to poor stores of fat beneath the skin and are a common physical symptom of malnutrition.

Fine hair on face (lanugo)

You might suddenly notice fine hair growth on your arms, cheeks, or back. This is called "lanugo," which is the body's attempt to conserve heat. It's a sign of malnutrition and will go away during nutritional rehabilitation.

Bloating

Bloating is one of the most common complaints we hear across all ED diagnoses. This can also occur when an individual is beginning to eat more consistently, but your metabolism (your body's engine, which includes the operation of all major organs and your gastrointestinal system) is still sluggish. Eating more will help speed up your metabolism, which will ultimately help reduce constipation, gas, and bloating.

Heart racing, chest pain

Some may feel pain in their chest or a racing heartbeat. The heart may speed up or slow down when changing positions as the heart works hard to pump blood to different organs. This can happen when the body is malnourished and/or during episodes of bingeing, periods of anxiety, or stress, exercise, dehydration, and many other situations. Consult with a doctor to get an expert set of eyes on what's happening in your body. An EKG (electrocardiogram) may be necessary as well.

Body

Body checking

Body checking is when someone repeatedly checks the parts of their body with which they are dissatisfied. This might be pinching your arm or belly, comparing yourself to old pictures, holding your wrist to see if its circumference has changed, or trying on many different pairs of jeans to feel which have gotten tighter or looser. Body checking can increase anxiety, depression, and body dissatisfaction.[13] A goal of treatment is to assess how often these behaviors occur and to stop them. Nothing positive comes out of body checking; most feel worse afterward. For more on this topic, see chapter 18.

Increased focus on body weight and shape

Body image dissatisfaction occurs when there is an intense preoccupation with one's size, shape, and body. This dissatisfaction underlies many EDs. Many pinpoint adolescence as the time when they began experiencing body image dissatisfaction. Adolescence is characterized by rapid emotional and physical growth, framed by puberty. By the end, most can hardly recognize their bodies anymore. The same might be true during pivotal life stages like pregnancy and menopause, where the body is undergoing many hormonal changes. Obsession and preoccupation with one's body can be concerning and can occur at any age.

Cognitive Function and Mood/Mindset

Obsessive thinking

EDs are often characterized by obsessions and preoccupations with food, weight, and shape. Obsessive thinking worsens with weight loss. Someone with an ED may count calories, track their meals on apps, and spend most of the day thinking about food, weight, or shape. Many admit this is exhausting. Obsessive thinking can turn into irrational and dangerous thinking. Obsessive tracking, counting, or goal setting can inevitably lead to heightened anxiety, as those suffering may or may not be able to stick with these often unattainable and dangerous goals. Someone suffering from an ED may begin to talk about how many calories they need to burn in order to eat. ("If I eat nine hundred calories today, then I have to burn nine hundred calories.") Doing so fails to consider that your body is burning far more than what a certain "machine" or "tracking device" might be reporting. The human body burns calories when digesting food (thermic effect), during sleep, and at rest.

Avoidance of social situations

Avoiding communal meals is common when an ED occurs. Social situations can be challenging for those who struggle with their relationship with food. Ordering from a menu can be overwhelming, especially while being expected to hold a social conversation. Eating in front of others or having food prepared by others in unknown portions can increase anxiety. Plus, being around alcohol can be tricky for some. A person may decide to skip social events to avoid having to "deal with food."

Mood changes: more depressed, anxious, irritable

We see an increase in irritability, depression, and anxiety as one reduces their food intake. You might notice you are fighting more with your loved ones, quickly losing your temper, or getting frustrated more easily, feeling more depressed, and/or experiencing emotional waves. This can feel overwhelming. Some of these feelings may have predated the ED, whereas others may be exacerbated by and/or newly present because of the ED. You will read more about the benefits of involving a therapist and/or a psychiatrist in chapter 10.

Brain fog and decreased concentration

Many people report feeling foggy. An insufficient amount of nutrition, chaotic eating, or engaging in disordered eating behaviors can decrease energy, concentration, memory, recall, ability to focus, and interest in and engagement with work/school/life.

As you can see, there are many signs and symptoms associated with EDs and/or disordered eating. Some behaviors might feel benign, such as a newfound interest in health, and others might seem more concerning, like becoming increasingly restricted and limited by what you will and will not eat. A progressively narrowing diet is always a concern because it increases the likelihood that you are not getting enough nutrition to support your body.

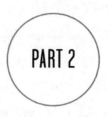

PART 2

The Plate-by-Plate Approach®

CHAPTER 3

Conducting Your Baseline Nutrition Assessment

Assessing Your Diet

Before implementing the Plate-by-Plate Approach®, it might be helpful to have an understanding of whether or not your ED has resulted in any nutritional deficiencies and of the ways the ED shows up when you're making food-related decisions. As you work through this chapter, the assessment tools and questions will guide you to focus on areas in which your diet is lacking and your ED is loudest. Some of these areas will be obvious to you (and perhaps to those around you). You might also discover a few areas that you didn't realize were an issue. This section will provide insight and ways to prioritize the fight against the ED when you feel ready.

We don't mean for this section to cause you shame but rather to illuminate trouble spots. It will help you identify where to start. Many of you might already be working with a dietitian who regularly assesses your diet and eating behaviors and coaches you on areas needing change. This book will augment your work. For those of you not working with a dietitian or treatment team, we hope this book motivates you to find a path forward.

Some of our patients have expressed, with a small dose of humor, that they feel "called out" by all the ways in which this assessment exposes their EDs. The first step of recovery is recognition; the ED will hide forever if you let it.

A Seven-Day Food Record

You can probably describe how you eat, what you eat, and what some of the "issues" are. But there is something very powerful about seeing your food reflected back to you on paper, meal after meal. We encourage you to keep a seven-day record: Log every breakfast, lunch, dinner, and snack. We don't want you to count calories, but do your best in recording food quantities.

Daily Food Record

MEAL	1	2	3	4	5	6	7
BREAKFAST							
SNACK							
LUNCH							
SNACK							
DINNER							
SNACK							

Food records can be a helpful tool for some but hard for others to use. Some patients have reported that it's stressful or triggering to keep a food record. If this is the case for you, please skip this part. You may be keeping food records in apps with your treatment team already. We will talk more about the use of apps and food records in chapter 10.

Assess Your Diet

VOLUME

How many days per week do you eat breakfast? Lunch? Dinner? Snacks? How many snacks per day do you typically eat?

Are there any times of day when you are eating larger amounts of food (bingeing or overeating)?

If you answered yes, are you noticing any patterns in your food intake before these episodes (for example, missed snack or meals)?

- When you eat, do you use a
  - » side salad or small plate,
  - » bowl,
  - » mug, or
  - » dinner plate (at least 10 inches in diameter)?
- When you eat, the plates are
  - » 100% full,
  - » 75% full,
  - » 50% full, or
  - » 25% full.

Assessment of volume

Are you missing meals or snacks throughout the week?

Are you using a 10-inch dinner plate?

Are your plates full?

VARIETY

Name foods and the number of servings you consume in each of the following categories. This will help you see if there are deficits in certain categories. There is more information about the benefits of each food group and the amounts recommended per day in chapter 5. We will explore more about foods you are specifically avoiding in chapter 15.

1. Grains/starches (e.g., bread, rice, cereal, pasta, potatoes)

2. Proteins (e.g., meat, poultry, fish, eggs, beans)

3. Fruits

4. Vegetables

5. Fats (e.g., butter, oil, avocado, nuts)

6. Dairy (e.g., milk, yogurt, cheese)

7. Snacks

Assessment of variety

Recall what your favorite meals used to be. Do you include these anymore?

Do you notice areas that are insufficient? If so, which need the most work?

Are you low in a specific food group? If so, which one(s)? Please list.

HYDRATION

Excess fluid consumption can have life-threatening consequences; too few can cause dehydration. Neither extreme is desirable, yet both are common in individuals with EDs. A rough estimate for how much fluid to take in is to consume half your body weight in fluid ounces. So if you are 200 pounds, the daily fluid recommendation would be 100 fluid ounces (this may come from water, milk, juice, coffee, tea, and some foods). Many of our patients don't wish to know their weight, so an alternative rule of thumb for reaching a sufficient level of hydration is to make sure your urine is a pale-yellow color throughout the day (think pale-lemonade color) but not too clear (like water). A concentrated apple juice urine color indicates you are dehydrated.

Dehydration is common in malnutrition and can cause dizziness and worsen orthostatic vital signs. It can be hard to stay on track with fluids, particularly for those taking certain medications, in certain climates (the sun can blunt the thirst mechanism) or altitudes, and for those with neurodiversity, where interoceptive awareness might be more difficult. Establishing a regular hydrating schedule, such as with each meal and snack or setting an alarm to hydrate, might be helpful.

Assessment of fluids

What are you drinking? List all drinks, including estimation of cups.

How is your hydration?

Do you think you are drinking enough?

Do you have a goal you want to set around hydration?

CAFFEINE

A total of 90 percent of adults consume caffeine, with the majority of consumption being from coffee (70 percent), cola drinks (16 percent), and tea (12 percent),[1] though the consumption of energy drinks has been on the rise.[2] There has also been a rise in caffeinated pre-workout supplements, energy drinks, chewing gum, gels, and other forms of caffeinated products in young adults and those involved in sports.[3] Many have wondered whether caffeine is dehydrating. Several studies have shown that caffeine consumption does not seem to impair overall hydration status or induce dehydration—it can, instead, help to contribute to a person's overall hydration status if their caffeine intake is mild.[4] Given that individuals with EDs may also be undernourished, medically compromised, or have unstable vitals, it is advised to discuss with your doctor or dietitian whether and how much caffeine you consume. In general, it is not advisable to drink large amounts of caffeine-containing products when struggling with an ED because caffeine can affect vital signs (heart rate, blood pressure, and orthostatic changes), appetite, and compliance with one's meal plan. Too much caffeine can make it difficult to obtain adequate nutrition, filling your stomach with liquids that may blunt your appetite, reduce adherence to the full meal plan, or suppress your appetite and alter your hunger and fullness cues (a trigger for bingeing when the caffeine wears off).

When consuming caffeine in high-heat and/or high-altitude settings, extra caution should be taken for those with EDs who may already be medically compromised; this increases the risk of dehydration, and vital signs and electrolyte abnormalities. Too much caffeine can alter the rhythm of the heart, cause jitteriness, increase anxiety and headaches, and cause significant sleep disruption.

The half-life of caffeine is 4 to 6 hours,[5] with caffeine metabolism varying per person. This means that if you have a caffeinated drink at

3:00 PM, roughly 25 percent of that caffeinated drink is still in your system at 3:00 AM. Many patients with EDs report having sleep concerns (insomnia or a delay in ability to fall or stay asleep). Assess how much caffeine you are consuming and when. You may want to make adjustments.

Assessment of caffeine intake

Have you checked with your doctor about whether you can have caffeine?

How many caffeinated drinks do you have per day?

- Coffee
- Tea
- Energy drinks
- Soda

How many caffeinated sports foods do you have per day?

- Gels
- GU Energy products
- Chewing gum
- Pre-workout products
- Sports supplements
- Pills

How would you describe your caffeine intake?

Is there a goal you want to set around hydration or caffeine?

Frequency of Eating Disorder Behaviors

To see where you are starting from, ask yourself the following questions.

Are you using food tracking apps? If yes, how do you feel about it/them?

Are you wearing an exercise watch or fitness tracker? If yes, how many and how do you feel about it?

Are you restricting? If yes, how often?

Are you bingeing? If yes, how often?

What are your triggers?

Are you purging? If yes, how often?

What are your triggers?

Are you using laxatives? If yes, how often?

What are your triggers?

Are you using diet pills? If yes, how often?

What are your triggers?

Are you exercising in a compulsive way? If yes, how often?

What are your triggers?

Assessment of eating disorder behaviors

What do you notice about your ED behaviors?

Which behaviors do you wish to target?

CONDIMENT USE AND/OR USE OF SWEETENERS

We often see our patients using excessive amounts of noncaloric sweeteners and interesting combinations of condiments that were not occurring before the onset of the ED. Researchers have also confirmed a prevalence of sweetener use, chewing gum, and diet soda.[6] This could be a sign of appetite abnormalities and/or undernutrition. The body seems to be seeking flavor, maybe as an attempt to obtain more food. And while these behaviors are consistent with a desire to avoid calories, they also indicate a desire for flavor.

Ask yourself the following questions.

Am I using an excessive amount of sweeteners?

Am I using more hot sauce, ketchup, mustard, etc., than most would consider to be typical? Has this changed since the onset of the ED?

Assessment of use of condiments and sweeteners

What, if anything, have you noticed about your relationship with sweeteners and condiments?

SLEEP

The recommended amount of sleep for adults is 7 to 9 hours per night, with more sleep required for athletes. Sleep affects mood, mental health (depression, anxiety, irritability), sports performance, reaction time,[7] split-second decision making,[8] injury risk,[9] academics, concentration, and more![10] Sleep can often be disrupted while in recovery from an ED, yet consistent sleep is vital to physical and emotional healing.

Assessment of sleep

How many hours of sleep are you getting per weeknight?

How many hours of sleep are you getting per weekend night?

Summary of Nutrition Assessment

Following is a chart that summarizes your findings from this chapter. Consider what items are most important to you to address.

CATEGORY	COMMENT
Food Volume	How is your food volume? Are you missing any meals and snacks?
Variety	What favorite foods, if any, are missing from your diet? What food groups are insufficient or missing from your diet?
Eating Disorder Behaviors	Which areas need the most work?
Hydration	How is your hydration?
Caffeine	How is your caffeine intake?
Substance Use	Are you using/abusing substances? Is your substance use impacting your nutrition?
Condiment/Sweetener Use	Are you using an excessive amount of condiments or sweeteners?
Sleep	Are you getting enough sleep?

CHAPTER 4

Achieving the Plate

THE **PLATE-BY-PLATE APPROACH**® is a no-numbers, no-measuring visual approach to refeeding. This approach provides a seamless transition to normal eating and a sense of relief, as it allows you to leave your measuring cups, tracking apps, and food scales behind. In this chapter you will find detailed steps to implement it successfully.

A Note About Anxiety

As you start your recovery, you might find that your anxiety level escalates. We encourage you to take a moment as often as you need, put the book down, and take five deep breaths. Then remember why this work is important to you.

Step 1: Choose a 10-Inch Plate

Okay, let's get started. The actual plate you use is critical in the Plate-by-Plate Approach®. Since this is a visual approach, it relies on a simple dinner-size plate as its backbone to ensure you have enough food. This is the only tool you will need to master this approach—no measuring cups or measuring spoons required! The plate size we recommend is roughly 10 inches wide.

The ED often loves to take shortcuts, and salad plates, toddler plates, paper plates, and plastic plates are generally too small to ensure you are being sufficiently nourished. The best plates are smooth, without ridges or inner circles. If you were only to fill the "inner circle," the volume provided would likely be insufficient. Here is an example of a plate design to avoid.

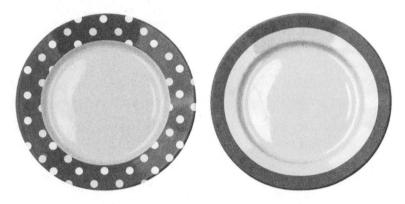

Those who use these "inner circle" plates inevitably fill the plate only to the inner circle, and eat less food. You can ultimately choose to use whatever plate you want (small plate, inner circle plate) and work your way up to the 10-inch plate, but we recommend starting with the full dose of medicine that we know works best to fight the ED.

This is a better plate.

The ED often prefers to eat out of a bowl, which is to be differentiated from one's cultural traditions. We have chosen a 10-inch plate so there can be full transparency about what is on your plate and to ensure it's "enough." It is hard to do that as easily from a bowl. The ED tends to love secrecy, which can be done more easily from a bowl. Many will take small bowls, which can result in small portions.

What Size Plate Are You Using?

Many wonder how to use the Plate-by-Plate Approach® with different plate sizes. When a 10-inch dish is not an option, here are a few tips to help you plate your meal adequately.

1.   If the plate is larger than 10 inches, it's okay to leave some blank space. Just make sure all 5 food groups are represented and the plate is mostly full.

2.   If the plate is smaller than 10 inches, really fill that plate with all 5 food groups (to the edges) and consider adding a drink or a dessert. Most likely, going back for second helpings will help meet your needs. Expect to see this when using paper plates, at parties or events.

3.   For plates that aren't round but are roughly 10 inches, fill them the same way you would a round plate.

Step 2: Choose a Plate Breakdown

The next step is to choose which plate breakdown is right for you. When choosing your plate, it is important to factor in your unique nutritional goals. Here, we are intentionally not using numbers. This is because the ED loves to get caught up and lost in numbers. The intention of this approach is to guide you, alongside your treatment team, to the right plate and overall plan for your needs.

Here, we have two plates from which you can choose.

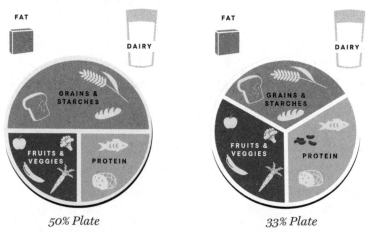

50% Plate   *33% Plate*

50% plate

This plate comprises 50% grains/starches, 25% protein, 25% fruits or vegetables, plus added fat and dairy or dairy alternative.

Who is this plate best for?

This plate is best for active adults who are engaging in moderate exercise (4 to 5 days per week, for 45 minutes or more), those who require weight restoration (teens or adults), athletes (teens or adults), anyone who is pregnant or breastfeeding, anyone with high nutritional needs due to a medical condition or medication or circumstance, or anyone eating intuitively. Note that the 50% plate will be a weight maintenance plate for some people, depending on body size, energy expenditure, and nutrition goals.

Body size plays a role as well. Those in larger bodies require more food, not less, contrary to what diet culture likes to tell you. This means that those in larger bodies likely will require the 50% plate or else could consider using the 33% plate paired with more frequent and denser snacks to meet their needs.

33% plate

This plate comprises 33% grains/starches, 33% protein, 33% fruits or vegetables, plus added fat and dairy or dairy alternative.

Who is this plate best for?

This plate is best for adults doing light exercise programs (1 to 3 days per week, 10 to 45 minutes), those struggling with purging and looking for a smaller volume to work toward keeping food down, or those who are not yet able to use the 50% plate. This plate is great for anyone eating intuitively. This plate may also be appropriate for children and younger adolescents.

Factors that affect plate choice

Age

Older adults: Nutrition needs decrease with age.

Adults: May start with the 33% plate but might need more food based on other factors (biological sex, activity, goals, body size). Biological sex and body size impact metabolic requirements. Biological males and those in larger bodies generally have higher energy needs.

Teens: Many teens and young adults need the 50% plate.

Exercise

Nutritional needs vary by duration, intensity, and frequency of one's exercise program.

- Lower-intensity exercise, duration, and frequency (walking, Pilates, yoga, stretching, light cycling for about 30 to 45 minutes) may use the 33% plate, while adding more snacks on days when exercising a little longer.

- Higher-intensity exercise, duration, and frequency (cyclists, runners, team sports, endurance sports, triathlon training, multi-sporting events) likely require the 50% plate, with additional snacks and/or the Accelerated Plate (see chapter 6).

Goals

Nutrition needs vary based on whether you are looking to maintain weight or restore weight. Weight loss is not compatible with ED recovery. That might be hard to come to terms with, but focusing on caloric restriction feeds the ED and perpetuates ED behaviors. Here are additional guidelines for goals—and while there may be exceptions, these guidelines are generally true.

- Those looking to gain weight, will likely need the 50% plate or the Accelerated Plate.

- Those looking to maintain weight may need the 33% plate, but this can vary. All factors listed above should be carefully considered (especially exercise).

- Those looking to reduce purging may benefit from following the 33% plate initially, simply to work on reducing purging episodes. Once purging is reduced, transition to the plate that best fits your needs.

Additional factors
- Extra food is needed for those who are pregnant or breastfeeding, those who are post-surgery, injured, or have high metabolic needs.

Examples
- A 30-year-old who is weight restored, exercising less than 3 times per week for 30 minutes, might be able to use the 33% plate.

- A 65-year-old who needs to gain weight for treatment with anorexia and is not exercising would need the 50% plate.

- An adult who is exercising 6 times per week for 2 hours a session, might be able to use the 50% plate.

- An adult in a larger body, looking for weight maintenance, who walks 1 hour, 4 times per week, might use the 50% plate.

How will I know this plate is working?

As you do this work, you will want to know whether you have chosen the right plate. Ask yourself the following questions.

- Am I meeting my goals? This might include gaining weight, if indicated, restoring vital signs, improving metabolism, and restoring hormonal balance. To be sure, check with a medical provider to see if, in fact, these areas are improving.

- Am I eating more consistently? This might be eating more regular meals and snacks than you were before.

- Have my binge episodes lessened in frequency?

- Is my mood and energy improving? You might feel more grounded, experience less brain fog, more energy, and more mental clarity. Note that increasing food may increase anxiety in the beginning, but that is to be expected!

- Is my relationship with food improving? Increasing the size, frequency, and variety in meals is a gateway to improving one's relationship with food.

Your nutritional needs are unique. While this self-assessment will help you get started, we advise that you also consult with a registered dietitian (RD) and your treatment team to ensure success and safety along the way.

Step 3: Include All the Food Groups

The Plate-by-Plate Approach® will help you to plate balanced meals. No matter which plate you choose to start with, include all 5 food groups: (1) grains/starches, (2) protein, (3) vegetables or fruits, (4) fats, and (5) dairy or a dairy alternative.

What does this look like? Let's say you're making chicken for dinner. That covers the protein section of the plate. What will your starch be? Pasta? Potatoes? Rice? A salad could be your vegetable that night, and salad dressing could be the fat. Add a cup of milk, and all food groups are represented. This plate is inclusive for those following a gluten-, dairy-, or allergen-free diet. Simply swap in the foods your body tolerates in each food category. We will cover much more about these food groups and the breakdown of the plate ratios in the next chapter.

Food group checklist

A checklist can be helpful when thinking about meal preparation and grocery shopping to ensure that all food groups are represented at each meal.

FOOD GROUP	FOOD ITEM AT MEAL
GRAINS/STARCHES	
PROTEIN	
VEGETABLE OR FRUIT	
FAT	
DAIRY OR DAIRY ALTERNATIVE	

Q: I make a lot of one-pot meals. How do those represent each food group?

A: Foods that have many of the food groups mixed in, like casseroles or Crockpot meals, can be plated using this approach as well. Here, the plate will be a combination of food groups. Think about which sections of the plate your dish takes up. If it's a mixed dish like chicken and broccoli, fill up enough of the plate so it covers both the protein and vegetable section. Then add the starch. A casserole like meat lasagna will cover most of the plate since all the food groups are in the dish. Then you might want to add something else, perhaps a side salad, to fill up the rest of the plate.

Step 4: Fill the Plate Up!

Now that you're clear on plate size and the recommended proportions of food groups, the next step is to make sure the meal is "enough." To follow this approach completely, *there should be no empty space left on the plate.* That is the ultimate goal, which might feel hard for you, but if the meal covers only 60 or 75 percent of the plate, there is likely not enough food to support your needs. It's possible to have all 5 food groups on the plate but not have enough. Here is a plate that has all the food groups (with milk on the side, not pictured) yet isn't full.

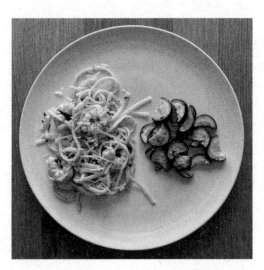

You may be thinking, *If I haven't eaten a full plate of food in a long time, shouldn't I start smaller?* Many years ago, it was common to increase the volume of food more slowly. Newer research shows that it is safe (and recommended) to start with calorically dense meals and an overall higher-calorie meal plan right away.[1] A more rapid recovery is also associated with a more favorable prognosis.[2] Increasing volume is not only safe but also associated with a better long-term outcome.

That said, we know that change is hard and your journey is your own. Of course, you can proceed at your own pace in whatever way feels right to you. A completely full plate, plus snacks, may feel like a lot of food to you. There really is no "right" way. For those whose goal is weight restoration, the volume required during this process will be high. This means that you will need to eat much more than those around you. We suggest keeping your eye on your own plate.

Keep Your Eyes on Your Own Plate

Comparisons are common, but when they pertain to food they can be dangerous. People have different energy requirements, which vary based on such factors as height, weight, biological sex, activity level, age, and nutritional goals. If you are in recovery, depending on your medical status and diagnosis, may need to restore weight, making your nutritional needs higher than your peers' (even if you appear to have similar needs). Your food recommendations are customized to you, and copying someone else's eating pattern is like copying someone else's medication protocol. You wouldn't do *that*, would you?

Watching friends eat can be triggering, especially when you see your friends eating less than you. But maybe they ate less at lunch because they are intuitive eaters, and they had a few extra snacks that day. Or maybe they have an ED and/or have a poor relationship with food?

What's most important is that you do you. No one else could possibly be modeling what is exactly right for you. Ask yourself:

- What is right for me?
- Why am I interested in someone else's style of eating?
- Is that desire coming from a grounded place or a fear-based place?
- What do I feel I need more of? Less of?

What is your eating environment?

Often, our patients describe eating at their desk, on their laps, in their bedrooms, or in the car. They have a meal, but kind of wish they weren't having the meal. . . .

What if you were intentional about having the meal? Think "Yes, I need this food. I am nourishing my body."

If it's loud and chaotic around you, it might feel harder to digest your food and have a pleasant eating experience. Can you find a quiet place to eat peacefully? Would it feel different if you set the table? Played music? Lit a candle? Even if you are eating alone, you deserve to eat with intention.

For some, certain kitchen smells are aversive, and others struggle with misophonia, an extreme dislike of certain sounds,[3] such as the sounds of people chewing. Some might need to look for an alternative dining environment that feels more safe and tolerable. Leaving the traditional dining setting might be hard for your loved ones. But cultivating a safe space for you—free of chaos, distraction, smells, noise, with tools that calm you—music, and yes, even television, might be what you need to be successful at mealtime.

Step 5: Decide on How Many Meals and How Many Snacks

We recommend a baseline goal of 3 meals and 2 to 3 snacks a day. For some, 3 meals and 2 snacks might be a nourishing place for your body at this time. For others, you might need 3 meals and 3 or 4 snacks per day to keep up with increased energy requirements. Snacks are recommended for those with and without an ED—adults and kids alike!

Snacks help keep your metabolism ignited, your blood sugar stable, and your energy up all day. Snacks also help you meet your ED recovery goals, whether it's to stop bingeing, aid in weight restoration, boost heart rate, balance hormones like estrogen or testosterone, or improve bone density. Eating between meals provides energy and fuels your muscles, your mind, and your workouts, all while supporting your daily life. Snacks also prevent that ravenous feeling, aka, "getting hangry." A high hunger level causes you to eat quickly and impulsively, bypassing your ability to tune in to your inner wisdom of what your body might actually need. For those who participate in exercise, systematic fueling helps with recovery, which facilitates peak performance and helps to prepare the body for the next day's workout. Some may try to avoid snacks thinking they will "save calories." Yet, inevitably this can lead to overeating or feeling lethargic or irritable.

The size and number per day of the snacks will depend on your nutritional needs and unique goals. We are typically of the mindset that, at a minimum, 3 meals and 2 snacks per day is recommended for most people. The volume of the plates and size of the snacks can be adjusted. If you require weight restoration, are exercising daily, are in a larger body, or are pregnant or breastfeeding, be prepared to increase the size and frequency of these snacks. Your dietitian can help guide you in what's best for you. For example:

- If you're not currently having snacks, consider adding 1 to 2 snacks to start and work your way up to more snacks.

- If you're having 2 snacks, but they are small, begin by increasing the size of the snacks.

- If you're already having 2 snacks that each include at least two different food items, then you can either make those snacks larger, or add a third snack.

What is considered a snack? Using the Plate-by-Plate Approach®, we recommend pairing a couple of food groups to make a complete snack. This can be a combination of any food groups of your choice, and will increase as the meal plan increases. To improve variety, satiety, and caloric density, we ask that you not use two of the same food groups in one snack (like an "apple and banana" or "carrots and strawberries"). Ideally, a snack would consist of unique food groups, such as yogurt (dairy) and granola (grain) or cheese (dairy) and crackers (grain). Examples of good snack choices are provided in chapter 7. Snacks might be plated or taken to go. You might also ask yourself: What sounds good? What challenges the ED?

Mealtime Scheduling

Eating on a schedule can help ensure mealtime success. For those of you who have children, it can be helpful to feed yourself when you feed your kids. Kids need to eat often (as you know!), so instead of just prepping their food, try prepping extra for yourself and sitting with them to eat. They are most likely on a schedule similar to what we are recommending for you: breakfast, snack, lunch, snack, dinner, snack. So say it with us: When they eat, you eat.

For those without children, set up a schedule for yourself and try to stick to it.

Example of a Mealtime Schedule

7:00 AM	Breakfast
10:00 AM	Morning Snack
12:30 PM	Lunch
4:00 PM	Afternoon Snack
7:00 PM	Dinner
10:00 PM	Evening Snack

How Long Should It Take to Eat Meals and Snacks?

Our patients often tell us about a meal or snack taking hours to eat. While there is no "right" duration of time in which to eat a meal or snack, as someone is working toward ED recovery, setting guidelines and boundaries helps to contain the meal and prevent it from running into the next, which would make it impossible to stay on track.

We know this work is hard, but we encourage you to set a reasonable guideline for mealtimes to maximize the likelihood of staying on track. We typically recommend:

MEALS: 30 minutes

SNACKS: 15 minutes

If you don't finish on time, we suggest you add a supplement like Ensure, BOOST, or Kate Farms for the rest of the meal that is left until you can eat the whole portion. This serves as a metabolic placeholder. It allows your body to get used to the volume of food, but also quickly leaves the stomach, and digests easily.

Include a variety of foods

Variety is an essential component to the Plate-by-Plate Approach®. It is important that you include different breakfasts, lunches, dinners, and snacks. So many of our patients will say that they "just love oatmeal so much" or "love Rx Bars" and "that's all they want to eat." Rigidity can keep those with an ED stuck in the same patterns, because they are scared to try something different. This fear may arise because they deem another choice to be unhealthy or too processed or they are scared that "those types of foods" are unhealthy or will "make them fat." Fear of weight gain and associated "fatphobia" is stigmatizing and also keeps people stuck in their ED.

An essential part of recovery is rebuilding your relationship with food. This will require work to shift how you think about and experience certain foods. Using food exposures, you might try having cold cereal instead of oatmeal and discover that it feels okay after all—and with repeated exposures, anxiety levels decrease. It is *much easier* to eat the same foods over and over again, but that does not fight the ED. The end goal is for you to feel truly free to eat anything and be flexible and open to all foods. Those whose food choices remain restrictive struggle to attend parties, go on dates, travel, and more.

For the best variety, sprinkle different choices throughout your meals and throughout your day. Meal choices can vary, as can individual protein, starch, vegetable/fruits, fat and dairy choices. There might be more variety now than there ever was before the ED treatment, and that's great! Try different breakfast choices: breakfast burritos, waffles, smoothie bowls, pancakes, oatmeal, and cereal. Explore lunch and dinner options: sandwiches, wraps, panini, stir-fries, ramen, burgers, rice and beans, sushi. Rotate the proteins (chicken, beef, fish, ham, eggs, peanut butter) and starches (bread, rice, potatoes, quinoa, couscous) and fats (oils, dressings, hummus). It's fun to shop at different stores to find new snacks that might be interesting or to find new recipes that might be fun to make.

Step 6: Do a Final Review: How Does the Plate Look?

Use this last step as a final review of how the plate looks. You might also want to ask yourself, "Does the plate make sense?" Sure, it has all the food groups present, but do these foods go together? We have seen chicken served with oatmeal, or salmon with pretzels. It's hard to convey what "cohesive" means, since of course this can be subjective. A great way to think about this is, Would you serve this plate of food to your friend or to a guest in your house?

The following are some of the reasons that we see plates lacking cohesiveness.

- Checking off the food groups while plating, but not looking at the plate as a whole
- Limited preferences
- Limited food availability
- Lack of culinary skills
- Diet mindset: avoiding certain foods (breads/starches, proteins, fats) or following a diet
- Unsure how to make cohesive meals

You don't have to be a skilled chef to make cohesive meals, and you don't have to spend a lot of money assembling cohesive plates. Fighting against the diet mindset and expanding your food preferences will allow you to work on plating more varied and cohesive plates. Check our sample plates in chapter 7 and our Instagram @platebyplateapproach for more visual plate examples.

Below is a plate that does not make sense. It has tofu nuggets (protein), carrots (vegetables), cereal and milk (grains and dairy), and pistachios (fats). While all food groups are accounted for, they didn't quite go together. This meal could be more cohesive by swapping the cereal with milk for rice and adding a glass of milk. Similarly, if adding oil or butter was possible, we would suggest that instead of nuts, or adding ranch dressing or hummus as a dip with the carrots.

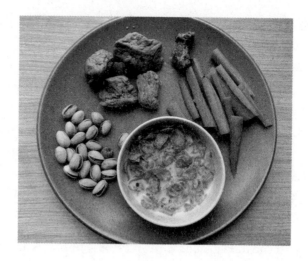

As you review your plate, ask yourself the following questions.

- Are all food groups present? Grains/starches? Protein? Fruit or vegetable? Dairy/dairy alternative? Fat?

- Is the plate 50% grains/starches, 25% protein, 25% fruit or vegetable? Or 33% grains/starches, 33% protein, 33% fruit or vegetable?

- Is the whole plate full?

- Does the meal "make sense" and feel cohesive?

- Have you challenged yourself?

We hope you find the Plate-by-Plate Approach® easy to follow and that it serves as a useful guide for your recovery journey.

CHAPTER 5

Why This Plate Breakdown?

WE ARE INUNDATED with nutrition information from a very young age, and it's nearly impossible to sort through the plethora of science (and pseudoscience) available at our fingertips. As you scroll through social media, watch TV, or listen to the radio, you'll likely see and hear messages touting the latest fad diet or weight-loss plan. You might read posters on the walls of your doctor's office encouraging you to "limit added sugar" or "eat more plant-based foods" or "fill half your plate with fruits and vegetables," and you may feel confused or overwhelmed.

Many of those messages are generalized nutrition recommendations and not specific to your quest to fight back against the ED. In fact, most of those messages actually work *against* recovery, as they tend to align with a diet mindset and often side with the ED. When the ED hears "limit sugar," it immediately thinks, "great, thanks, I will" and swears off desserts and baking for eternity—rather than working on exposures to decrease anxiety around food. Or when hearing "eat more fruits and vegetables," the ED hears permission to take less food, which can lead to prolonging the illness, a greater preoccupation with food, and potential bingeing.

With the Plate-by-Plate Approach®, we aim to simplify, so that you can build balanced yummy meals and snacks based on your unique needs, while fighting back against the ED. In this chapter, we break down each food group to help clarify its important role and provide examples of foods in each food group.

Grains and Starches

Grains and starches are rich sources of carbohydrates, one of three macronutrients the body requires for basic functioning (the others are protein and fat). Carbohydrates can be found in multiple food groups (grains/starches, fruits, and dairy or dairy alternatives) and provide necessary energy to every cell in the body. Carbohydrates are the most important source of fuel for your brain, heart, and muscles, yet we often hear patients saying that "carbs make them bloated" or wondering if they should "cut out carbs." Much of this dialogue has come from diet culture, which has stigmatized carbohydrates through popular fad diets like Atkins, South Beach, and the Keto Diet, to name a few. The antidote to the fear around these foods is the inclusion of a variety of carbohydrate-rich foods. Repeated experiences with these foods reduces anxiety and builds confidence in how your body responds to these foods, once fully nourished.

Unfortunately, living in and navigating a carbohydrate-phobic world can be tricky. It's almost impossible to avoid messages telling us to "limit processed or white carbohydrates" or to "eat more whole grains." The reality, however, is that carbohydrates are essential. Our brain runs on glucose, which is really just sugar (or carbohydrate) in its simplest form! Glucose is digested from the carbohydrate foods we consume, enters the bloodstream, and is stored in our liver and muscles for later use. To obtain enough glucose for the brain and all other cellular function, carbohydrates must be included in meals and snacks throughout the day.

Carbohydrate requirements vary from one individual to the next; the Institute of Medicine (IOM) set an acceptable macronutrient distribution range (AMDR) for carbohydrates of 45 to 65 percent of total calories.[1] This is why we recommend filling one third to one half of your plate with grains/starches to ensure you're getting enough carbohydrates to meet your body's needs.

To ensure that plating grains/starches is simple and adequate, we encourage you to consider only grains and starches for this category (bread, rice, pasta, cereal, potatoes) rather than mixing in different carbohydrate foods (like fruit, dairy/dairy alternatives). This will help you get the right balance of foods on your plate, fill the plate with an adequate volume of food, and keep things simple. For more examples of foods in the grains/starches category, see the table on page 76.

Carbohydrates: Fuel For Sports

Carbohydrates are central to sports performance, especially before, during, and after training. Carbohydrates are fundamental for maintaining sufficient glycogen levels, which is your body's "energy tank." Before a workout, carbohydrates along with some protein are recommended to provide your body with energy to sustain your workout. For example, some pre-workout options might include a banana and a yogurt, a granola bar and fruit, or trail mix and apple juice. When exercise lasts over an hour and is intense, it is recommended that easily digestible carbohydrates be added during your workout. This can be something like a GU, gel, or a sports drink. After practice, it's important to recover by refueling with mostly carbohydrates and some protein. Examples might be a smoothie, chocolate milk and a protein bar, or by having a meal. Without adequate carbohydrates, a person might experience fatigue, sluggishness, decreased endurance, difficulty recovering, brain fog, and trouble concentrating. Quite literally, there will not be enough gas in your tank to perform at whatever you are trying to do: your sport, your job, your life.

Variety is key

Throughout this process, try to add a variety of carbohydrates to all your meals and snacks. We often see repetitive breakfasts, for example, an oatmeal bowl every day or the same quinoa served for dinner every night. The same foods just might be keeping the ED alive and breathing beneath the surface.

It's important to vary your carbohydrates to include both whole grain *and* non–whole grain starches. Non–whole grains, as in . . . white starches? Yes. Here is why. When you eat out, the breadbasket *is almost never whole grain.* It's important that you can eat regular bread!

While whole grains objectively do provide more fiber, protein, and B vitamins than their refined counterparts (think brown versus white rice), eating too much of them can cause digestive discomfort. EDs already cause a lot of gastrointestinal distress—we don't want to make it worse! Whole grains contain the "bran" part of the grain, which is the hard or fibrous outer layer of grains like rice, wheat, and barley. Fiber plays an important role in moving food through the digestive tract, but in malnourished individuals the digestive tract tends to slow down. Too much fiber can worsen constipation, bloating, and gas. It's a little like a traffic jam in your intestines: If the road is at a standstill, adding more cars (or in this case, fiber) won't make the traffic clear; it will make it worse. Variety helps keep things moving without overwhelming your digestive tract.

What about gluten sensitivity? Gluten is a protein found in wheat, rye, and barley, giving these grains their chewy texture and strong structure once processed. Many individuals claim to be gluten sensitive or intolerant because they're experiencing digestive discomfort such as gas and bloating. Research suggests that about 6 percent of the US population is gluten intolerant. It's more common than celiac disease, which affects about 1 percent of the population.[2] If you're concerned that you are gluten intolerant or sensitive, or if you think you may have celiac disease, we recommend consulting your doctor, who may suggest a referral to a gastroenterologist for additional screening. If you do have celiac disease and need to eliminate gluten from your diet, it's still possible to meet the grain/starch recommendations of the Plate-by-Plate Approach® by including gluten-free substitutions such as rice, potatoes, and corn-based products.

If you do not have celiac disease, the next question is whether the gluten sensitivity and the onset of the ED coincide. If so, it is possible that gluten was removed as a widely accepted form of food restriction, cleverly masking the ED. That may be hard to tease apart, so we suggest food exposure. Rather than restricting foods you are concerned may be at the root of bloating, gas, or stomach pain, try including them as part of your meals or snacks to see if, once renourished, your body can tolerate them again. Malnutrition often leads to digestive discomfort. Rather than blaming (and subsequently removing) the foods you eat, improving nutrition and including a wide variety of foods will restore gut health.

Protein

Found in almost every tissue in the body, protein is an essential building block. Dietary protein is made up of amino acids, little building blocks that make up the bigger protein structure. There are animal- and plant-based sources of protein, and both contain amino acids. Animal forms of protein (meat, poultry, fish, eggs, dairy) contain the complete combination of amino acids necessary to build and repair tissue in the body, whereas plant-based proteins (beans, legumes, nuts) require complementary proteins (grains) to complete the amino acid chain required to build and repair tissue.

There are many myths surrounding protein, such as "more protein is better" or that "eating more protein yields bigger muscles." On the contrary, the body has a minimum protein requirement and additional protein isn't utilized to build more muscle, it's stored as energy instead. Strength athletes like bodybuilders do need more protein than endurance athletes, but some don't realize that they also need a significant amount of carbohydrates, calories, and fats to support their weight gain and muscle-building goals. Sufficient fuel, being at an appropriate weight for your body, and consuming a balanced diet will ensure that hormones such as estrogen and testosterone are in the normal range. Too much protein has a high-satiety factor and can often sabotage one's efforts in staying consistent with their meal plan, especially as it pertains to ED recovery wherein energy requirements can be two to three times one's baseline. We often see patients try to gain weight by adding protein shakes, protein bars, and even "mass gainer shakes," but these often backfire, making it hard to finish out the day on track with your meal plan.

Protein Powder

If you are choosing to use a supplement like a protein powder, we recommend that the supplement be NSF certified,[3] Informed Choice or third-party tested. Third-party testing and certification status ensures that the supplement contains the ingredients listed on the label, is not contaminated (heavy metals, herbicides, pesticides), and does not contain banned substances.[4] Both Informed Choice and NSF offer downloadable apps so you can see what products are available and whether your product is certified.

Most American adults are eating approximately twice the recommended amount of protein per day.[5] Eating enough protein is fairly easy to accomplish, when you consider protein is so readily available in foods such as chicken, turkey, eggs, fish, beans, tofu, dairy products, nuts, and even grains like quinoa and pasta.

A plate that is about 25% protein is adequate to meet the needs of most adults, especially considering one's total protein intake includes protein from food groups like the aforementioned dairy and grains. The average minimum amount of protein required for an adult can be met by filling 25% to 33% of your plates with foods containing protein. Those in larger bodies and those who are athletes involved in strength training have higher needs.

For a nonathlete, a sample breakfast that is adequate in protein might include two slices of buttered bread, two eggs, a glass of milk, and fruit. This breakfast example makes up greater than one third of the daily protein needs for a nonathlete. Add 2 more meals that are similar in protein content and 2 to 3 snacks that include some protein and the nonathlete will have easily consumed enough protein that day.

What about vegetarian and vegan plates? For lunch, a vegetarian might have a bean, rice, and cheese burrito with guacamole and a dressed side salad. A vegan might have that same lunch with vegan cheese instead of dairy cheese. These plates provide greater than 50 percent of daily protein needs from lunch alone. So, you can see that it's not difficult to meet daily protein needs when following the Plate-by-Plate

Approach® and filling 25% to 33% of each plate with a protein-rich food. That is, assuming you are eating enough volume to meet your energy needs and consume a variety of nutrients. If you're concerned about meeting your protein requirements, we suggest consulting a non-diet registered dietitian (a dietitian that focuses on health behaviors, not weight loss or dieting).

While it may be easy on paper to fill 25% of your plate with protein, we also understand that protein-rich foods might increase anxiety or be difficult to include. Consider what might be long-standing food preferences and what might be connected to the ED. Simply put: Is your ED showing up in the choices you have made around which proteins you are consuming? For example, if you are a vegan or a pescatarian: Is that who you really are, or is that something the ED has created?

Another consideration for those following a vegetarian or vegan diet is iron content. Low iron levels may cause you to feel tired, weak, or irritable. Iron comes in two forms, heme and nonheme iron. Heme iron is found in animal proteins and nonheme iron is found in plant sources like beans, cereals, nuts, and chocolate. If you have concerns, please check with your doctor to assess iron levels, including checking your ferritin level (storage form of iron). Those at risk for iron deficiency, which would also include those with heavy menstrual cycles, should take a daily multivitamin. Vegetarians and vegans will want to add a multivitamin to ensure adequate intake from vitamins and minerals that may be lacking in the diet (e.g., B12 and iron).

Fruits and Vegetables

It's no secret that fruits and vegetables are jam-packed with vitamins, minerals, antioxidants, and fiber, but there is such a thing as eating too many of them. We often see plates that are filled high with fruits and vegetables. Our patients admit that despite the "healthy" appearance of their food, they know their diet is insufficient. Fruits and vegetables are important for gastrointestinal health, reducing inflammation in the body, preventing disease, keeping the immune system healthy, and many other reasons. You can reap these benefits by filling your plate with approximately one fourth fruit or vegetables. Too many fruits/vegetables compete with other more calorically dense foods and contribute to digestive discomfort, including premature fullness, gas, diarrhea, and even acid reflux.

Individuals who struggle with food volume should consider limiting this group to cooked, pureed, soft, dried, or juiced versions of fruits and vegetables to lower the overall food volume on the plate. To maximize the nutritional content of this food group, consider varying the type and color of fruits/vegetables on the plate from one meal or snack to the next. The greater the variety, the more vitamins, minerals, and antioxidants provided. There is also research that shows that variety in plant foods helps to support the microbiome and gut health.[6]

Some individuals who eat excessive amounts of fruits/vegetables may notice a yellow/orange tint to their hands and possibly the whites of their eyes. With darker-pigmented skin tones, this can be harder to spot. If this sounds like it could be you, you might compare your palms with those of a friend or family member. A slightly orange hue in your palm could indicate hypercarotenemia—an excessive buildup of beta-carotene in the body resulting from overconsumption of carotenoid-containing foods (carrots, red peppers, sweet potatoes, kale, etc.) in the absence of a varied diet. Hypercarotenemia is not dangerous but can be a warning sign that the diet is unbalanced and may be lacking in variety and overall caloric density. Reducing high beta-carotene foods while shifting the balance to a plate that is 33% to 50% grains/starches, 25% protein, and only 25% fruits/vegetables will improve this condition and normalize skin color. As your nutrition improves, you will look less orange over time.

There will be times when the vegetables might not be separated on the plate. Vegetables might be found in sauces, soups, and as part of the meal in certain traditional cuisines. For example, Indian food is well-known for pureeing vegetables as part of their curries. If the vegetable is part of the sauce, consider that your veggie for the meal but make sure your plate has sufficient volume.

What If I Hate Fruits and Vegetables?

"If one raspberry is moldy, I have to throw the whole container out; it's gross," one adult patient told us. "Even the thought of eating vegetables makes me gag," said another. How can you follow the Plate-by-Plate-Approach® when this happens? If this sounds like you, consider making a list of fruits and/or vegetables that you can tolerate. Consider whether a different preparation method would help. Are soft, cooked vegetables easier to eat or raw crunchy ones? Do you prefer fruit blended in a smoothie or in juice form? What about purees like applesauce or dried fruit like raisins or apricots? Maybe you only like one or two vegetables (baby carrots and tomato sauce—yes, that still counts as a vegetable). Or you don't like whole oranges, but you'll happily drink orange juice. No matter your preference, start by including on the plate or on the side the fruits and veggies that you do like. Over time, work on exposure to new or different forms of fruits and vegetables as you would any other food group.

You should also consider what are lifelong preferences versus ED preferences. If you have always disliked fruits and veggies but have a few that you regularly include, you may not need to change anything unless you want to. If, however, you have cut out roasted veggies for a fear of oli, or fruit juice because you heard it's "too high in sugar," that is something to work on including in your diet again. That way, the ED doesn't hijack your ability to eat a wide variety of fruits and veggies.

In the short term, for someone who won't go near a fruit and will only eat vegetables (or vice versa), fill the section of the plate with whichever one you will eat. Over time, you can decide whether you want to work on exposures to expand your palate.

For individuals with ARFID, please refer to chapters 15 and 16 for additional information about food exposure and variety.

Fats: Added to Each Meal

Thanks to the low-fat craze of the 1980s and 1990s, fats have had a notoriously bad rap for decades. Americans were told to "consume less fat" for fear of "obesity" and heart disease. And yet, in subsequent decades we saw a sharp increase in rates of "obesity," heart disease, and later, type 2 diabetes. Food companies removed fats and replaced them with sugar and carbohydrates. So, instead of eating a balance of macronutrients (carbohydrates, proteins, and fats), Americans were eating mostly carbohydrates and proteins. Without fats, there was very little satiety (fullness), so it was easy to bypass the body's natural stopping place, and eat the whole box of SnackWell's. You never felt full! Fat-free foods do not have the same mouthfeel or pleasurable sensation that enables people to feel satisfied. All macronutrients are important and are essential ingredients in establishing your relationship with hunger and fullness.

For those with EDs, fat is commonly feared. It's calorically dense, often perceived as a "greasy" or "oily" food. It's commonly associated with foods that feel scary, such as fried foods. Perhaps the worry is as straightforward as "eating fat will make me fat." First, it's important to realize that one food does not have the ability to cause weight gain. Also, it's important to realize that fearing "fat" and living life to control weight keeps the ED alive. Size acceptance and working on dismantling fatphobia are important aspects of ED recovery work. Your fears around "becoming fat" are also offensive to those in larger bodies around you, implying that something is wrong with diversely shaped bodies.

Fats are an important aspect of meals and part of the preparation of foods (i.e., roasting potatoes in oil or adding coconut milk to curries). However, when foods are cooked in oil or fat, that fat is often cooked off during the cooking process and what remains is then divided among several servings. Therefore, the fat used in food preparation is generally not sufficient to meet individual needs for dietary fats. We recommend adding fats to the plate *after* cooking, even if fat was used during the cooking process. This means adding butter to bread even if you use oil to sauté the spinach on the plate. Fats can be found in a variety of foods such as oils, butter, hummus, avocado, nuts, seeds, ice cream, cookies, and chocolate.

What role do fats play in the body?

Dietary fats play vital roles in the body, including protecting your organs from damage. A concentrated source of energy, they help keep mealtime volume manageable. The human brain is nearly 60 percent fat, which is essential for the brain's function and ability to perform. Essential fatty acids are required for optimal health, but they cannot be synthesized by the body and must be obtained from dietary sources.[7] EFAs are made up of omega-3 fatty acids (found in fish, flaxseeds, chia seeds, and walnuts) and omega-6 fatty acids (found in canola, soybean, safflower, corn, and sunflower oils and in meat, poultry, and eggs).

Dietary fatty acids also make up a lipid bilayer in our cells and are an essential precursor for estrogen and testosterone synthesis. For individuals struggling with amenorrhea or low testosterone levels, adding fats back to the diet, along with weight gain, helps produce estrogen for biological females, which regulates periods, and boost testosterone for biological males. Fats are also essential to the absorption of fat-soluble vitamins A, D, E, and K.

For those struggling with binge eating, adding enough fats to meals and snacks can help regulate satiety, which in turn, prevents bingeing. Fats slow the rate of digestion and increase feelings of fullness.

Strategies for Adding More Fats to Your Diet

Breakfast

- Spread a nut butter (peanut, almond, etc.) on toast, an English muffin, or a bagel. Or mix a nut butter into oatmeal or add it to a smoothie.

- Sprinkle nuts on top of full-fat granola or mix them into oatmeal.

- Add avocado or guacamole to toast or breakfast burritos.

Lunch

- Use mayo on sandwiches.

- Add avocado or guacamole to sandwiches.

- Add hummus to sandwiches or on the side as a dip.

- Dip veggies in ranch dressing.

- Add a side that contains fat, such as a cookie, chocolate, trail mix, nuts, or chips.

- Add cheese (cheeses can be counted as fats if not already used as dairy, otherwise add an additional serving).

- Add seeds such as sunflower, pumpkin, or hemp.

Dinner

- Add additional oil after cooking (30 percent evaporates during the cooking process).

- Add butter or oil to bread, pasta, rice, or veggies.

- Add chips as a side.

- Cook with sauces that contain fat (for example, a cream or cheese sauce). Use salad dressing (salad should never be dry!).

- Sprinkle nuts, such as candied pecans or walnuts, and seeds onto salads.

- Add feta or goat cheese to a salad or sprinkle on top of veggies.

- Add avocado to a salad.

Dairy or Dairy Alternative: Added to Each Meal, or about 3 Servings Per Day

Calcium is a mineral used in bone formation and found in concentrated amounts in dairy foods. It plays an integral role in bone health and other body functions. Think of our bones as a storage bank for calcium. When we consume adequate amounts of dietary calcium, we don't dip into our "bone bank." When calcium content in the diet is inadequate, we withdraw calcium from that bank to spend on normal body functions like muscle contractions, maintaining a steady heart rhythm, and blood clotting. During childhood, adolescence, and young adulthood, peak bone mass is achieved through diet and exercise. There's some debate about when peak bone mass is achieved, but most researchers agree that

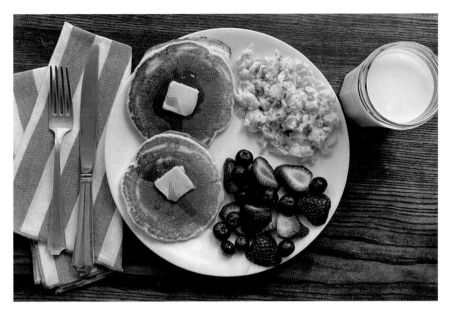

BREAKFAST 50% PLATE: *two pancakes (50% starch), scrambled eggs (25% protein), mixed berries (25% fruit), milk (dairy), butter (fat)*

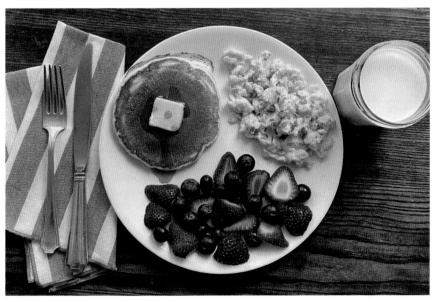

BREAKFAST 33% PLATE: *one pancake (33% starch), scrambled eggs (33% protein), mixed berries (33% fruit), milk (dairy), butter (fat)*

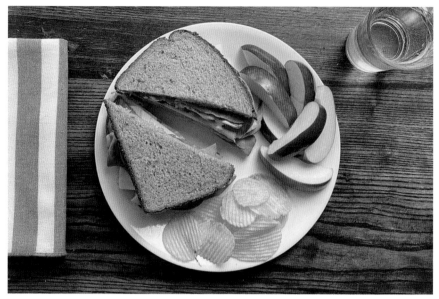

LUNCH 50% PLATE: *bread and chips (50% starch), turkey slices (25% protein), apple slices and lettuce (25% fruit/veg), cheese slices (dairy), mayo (fat)*

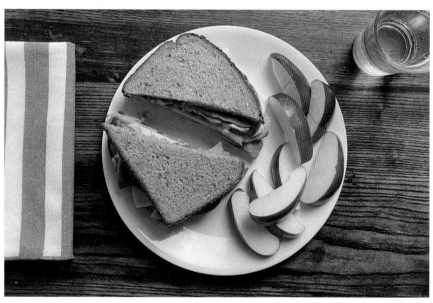

LUNCH 33% PLATE: *bread (33% starch), turkey slices (33% protein), apple slices and lettuce (33% fruit/veg), cheese slices (dairy), mayo (fat)*

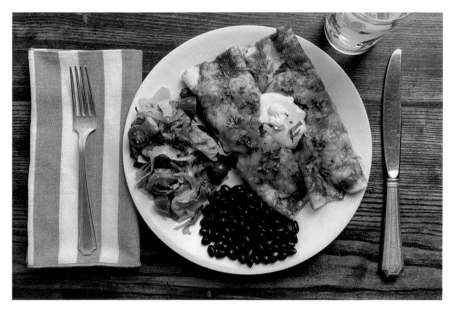

MEXICAN DINNER 50% PLATE: *two tortillas (50% starch), chicken enchilada filling and black beans (25% protein), salad (25% veg), cheese (dairy), sour cream (fat)*

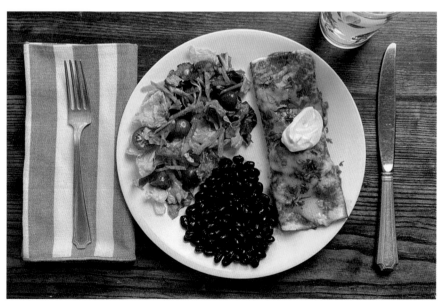

MEXICAN DINNER 33% PLATE: *one tortilla (33% starch), chicken enchilada filling and black beans (33% protein), salad (33% veg), cheese (dairy), sour cream (fat)*

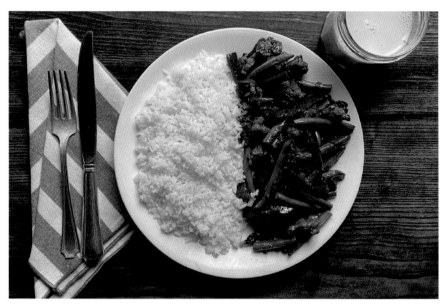

VEGAN/VEGETARIAN DINNER 50% PLATE: *rice (50% starch), seitan (25% protein), mixed vegetables (25% veg), soy milk (dairy), oil in stir-fry (fat)*

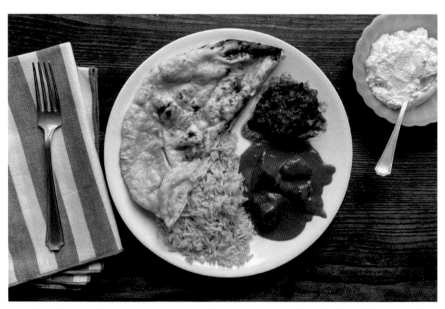

INDIAN DINNER 50% PLATE: *naan and rice (50% starch), chicken tikka masala (25% protein), vegetable fritter (25% veg), yogurt (dairy), oil in tikka masala (fat)*

it's somewhere between ages twenty-five and thirty-five.[8] After that, bone mass is no longer accrued and the bone bank is filled as much as it will ever be. It is essential to preserve the supply by consuming adequate calcium from food, maintaining good hormone levels (by eating enough to meet your needs), and doing weight-bearing exercises.

There are many sources of calcium. Dairy sources are well absorbed and utilized, since they are high in vitamin D and also contain fats. These include milk, yogurt, cheese, and kefir (probiotic drink). For some, milk may not be well tolerated, or liked, and people can turn to other sources to meet their needs. These include plant-based calcium sources, including tofu, almonds, soy, edamame, dark leafy greens, fortified juices, and cereals. High calcium greens include kale and spinach, however, it's important to note they also contain oxalates, making them less absorbable than other sources.

The Plate-by-Plate Approach® includes a source of dairy or a dairy alternative at each meal to ensure that individuals meet their recommended daily calcium needs, about 1,000 to 1,300 mg per day. One cup of milk, for example, contains about 300 mg calcium; 1 cup of yogurt contains about 450 mg calcium; and 1 ounce of cheddar cheese contains about 200 mg calcium. Three daily servings of dairy foods meet the majority of calcium needs. The rest is achieved through consumption of calcium-rich nondairy foods, such as grains, dark green leafy veggies, beans, nuts, tofu, fish, and others. Aiming for 3 servings per day (or 1 serving per meal) will provide almost all your daily calcium requirement.

Dairy is also a good source of vitamin D, and most dairy alternatives are fortified with vitamin D, which helps the body absorb and utilize calcium. Together, vitamin D and calcium help build and maintain strong bones.

Calcium is particularly important for those struggling with EDs, as many of our patients have suppressed hormones, which reduces bone density and increases the likelihood of fractures. For postmenopausal women and seniors, there is a greater risk of osteoporosis. Establishing regular periods in adolescence and early adulthood protects bones. As you age, however, estrogen will decline with the onset of perimenopause (or menopausal transition) and eventually menopause. During the menopausal transition period, the average reduction in bone mineral density (BMD) is about 10 percent, with some women losing up to 20 percent.[9] It is estimated that approximately one in ten women over the age of sixty worldwide are affected by osteoporosis, a disease that reduces BMD.[10] To preserve bone strength postmenopause, obtaining adequate dietary calcium and vitamin D is necessary. Calcium and vitamin D requirements increase as we age, but for women, the need for calcium specifically increases at age fifty-one (roughly the same time the average woman reaches menopause).

What if I'm lactose intolerant, vegan, allergic to dairy, keep kosher, or hate milk?

Some individuals are lactose intolerant, lactose sensitive, keep kosher, or allergic to dairy. If that's you, there are a number of ways to meet your body's needs. First, if you're lactose intolerant, you might try lactose-free versions of dairy products (available at most major grocery stores). You can also try using a lactase enzyme supplement. It adds lactase to your stomach to help break down the milk sugar lactose, which is responsible for digestive discomfort.

It's also not uncommon for digestive discomfort to be blamed on lactose sensitivity when the culprit isn't lactose. A malnourished body does not always produce sufficient digestive enzymes to break down food. That means you might never have been lactose intolerant or sensitive prior to the onset of the ED or a period of malnutrition, and then suddenly you're gassy, bloated, and uncomfortable when you eat dairy. The good news is, as you become better nourished, you will start making those enzymes again. The substitutes listed above can help until you are better nourished. It also may be the case that dairy was an "easy to restrict" food, because it's an accepted food intolerance in our society. In that case, we encourage you to challenge the ED and add real dairy foods back in. The greater the frequency of dairy exposures, the easier it will be to eat over time, and you will be practicing steps toward recovery.

Other options, for those of you who are vegan, allergic to dairy, keep kosher, or hate milk would be to try plant-based dairy-free milk alternatives. These are different from cow's milk, so if you dislike milk or never tolerated it, this might work for you. This will also work for those who keep kosher, where milk cannot be paired on your plate or eaten in conjunction with meat meals. You can include fortified oat, flax, soy, hemp, and pea protein milks. It may take time to become comfortable experimenting with these new options. Many of these plant-based milks offer flavors like vanilla and chocolate, so try them! We don't recommend almond or rice milk because they have very different nutrient profiles than dairy milk and tend to be too low-calorie.

Strategies for Getting More Dairy in Your Diet

Breakfast
- Add a glass of milk to drink or to use in cereal.
- Prepare oatmeal with milk instead of water.
- Include yogurt or cottage cheese.
- Serve kefir, a probiotic smoothie drink, on the side.
- Add cheese to scrambled eggs.
- Add portable cheese sticks or Babybel cheese on the side (remember to serve two, as these are lower-calorie options).
- Make a fruit smoothie with milk or yogurt.

Lunch
- Add a glass of milk or chocolate milk. Look for shelf-stable or individual-size boxes that don't require refrigeration and can be easily packed.
- Add cheese to sandwiches.
- Serve yogurt or kefir on the side.
- Crumble feta cheese or goat cheese over a salad.
- Use a spreadable cheese like Brie on sandwiches.

Dinner

- Add a glass of milk or chocolate milk.

- Add yogurt or kefir on the side.

- Top a stir-fry or cooked broccoli with shredded cheese.

- Add Parmesan cheese to pasta dishes.

- Melt cheese on bread or a tortilla.

- Crumble blue cheese or goat cheese over a salad.

- Add ice cream to the meal.

Common Foods by Food Group

STARCHES	PROTEINS	FRUITS AND VEGETABLES	DAIRY	FATS
White Pasta	Chicken	Apple	Whole Milk	Oil
Whole Wheat	Turkey	Orange	2% Milk	Butter
Pasta	Hamburger	Grapes	Lactaid Milk	Cream Cheese
White Rice	Steak	Bananas	Cheese	Salad Dressing
Brown Rice	Meatballs	Nectarine	Yogurt	Mayo
Yellow Rice	Swordfish	Plum	Smoothie with	Avocado
Quinoa	Halibut	Strawberries	Milk	Nuts
Couscous	Salmon	Blueberries	Kefir	Peanut Butter
Tortellini	Shrimp	Blackberries	Cottage Cheese	Almond Butter
Ravioli	Tilapia	Juice		Other Nut
Bread	Ham	Applesauce	*Dairy-Free*	Butters
Rolls	Roast Beef	Asparagus	*Alternatives:*	Hummus
Tortillas (Corn/	Peanut Butter	Broccoli	Soy Milk	
Flour)	Almond Butter	Salad	Pea Protein Milk	
Pita	Other Nut	Mushrooms	Oat Milk Yogurt	
Corn	Butters	Bok Choy		
Cereal	Tofu	Kale		
Oatmeal	Beans	Swiss Chard		
French Toast	Hummus	Green Beans		
Waffles	Dairy Foods			

———————

CHAPTER 6

Accelerated Nutritional Rehabilitation

FOR MANY RECOVERING from an ED, weight gain is necessary to achieve complete metabolic and psychological recovery. Some individuals have high metabolic needs, including athletes, those in larger bodies, and anyone requiring weight gain. This chapter is designed to help meet the nutritional needs for those requiring more than what the 50% plate (discussed in chapter 4) offers. Individuals requiring steady weight gain will have increased needs. For these individuals, we've designed the Accelerated Plate. This plate follows the same basic structure as the 50% plate, with adjustments and strategies to increase the volume of food it provides. For some, this plate will help with weight gain, and for others, this plate will support weight maintenance, since nutritional needs vary individually. We also talk through strategies for those of you who need to gain weight, and subsequent changes in the body that may occur. Some of you reading this might not need to gain weight, and those sections of this chapter might not apply.

Why Weight Gain May Be Difficult

Weight gain may be necessary for those who have lost weight, have low estrogen or testosterone levels or continue to have irregular or absent menstrual cycles, and for anyone with unstable vitals (low heart rate or orthostatic changes in pulse or blood pressure). Many people are surprised to hear that they need to gain weight as part of the journey to nourish themselves back to health. Weight gain can be necessary for older adults who might have spent their lives dieting and feel dumbfounded to now hear the message to "gain weight." Weight gain may be indicated for those in larger bodies in order for the brain, hormones, vital signs, metabolism, and relationship with food to improve. Those in a larger body may be overlooked in their need to gain back the weight lost due to diet culture's preference for smaller bodies, the weight stigma carried by clinicians working with these individuals, and the expectation that they "should" be at a lower weight. Clinicians need to be aware that serious medical complications can occur for those in all body shapes and sizes. Loved ones and partners might also feel surprised: "But she looks fine!" Or you might feel confused: "I'm not emaciated!" Remember, EDs can affect anyone, irrespective of how they look, and the treatment and correct "dose" of nutrition are important for a full, lasting recovery.

Many are shocked to learn they can eat *this much* while barely gaining any weight. The body desperately wants and needs this food. As you begin to add more fuel, your metabolism (your body's engine) starts working again to provide you more energy; to allow for an improvement in mood, vitals, and/or hormones; and to enable better temperature regulation. Your period may return! This is known as "metabolic recovery"—your metabolism is recovering and waking up. This is exciting, as many patients had come to us saying, "I messed up my metabolism with my eating disorder." But that's not true. The metabolism is resilient and can increase with consistent nutritional rehabilitation.[1] *Read that again*, because so many people worry that they have caused permanent damage to their metabolism.

The greater your intake of fuel, the more your body will use it. And so goes the process of restoring one's metabolism. This can be surprising to the ED, which has become accustomed to eating only small amounts. Now the body needs you to eat more to keep up with its faster metabolism. It's a beautiful thing.

Energy requirements for those who are malnourished, particularly for those who need to restore weight, are high. Often, as refeeding continues, the body can become hypermetabolic.[2] This means the metabolism speeds up faster than what is considered to be one's baseline. This increased metabolic rate increases your energy expenditure and calorie requirements, making weight gain more difficult. During refeeding, there is an increase in the thermogenic effect of food, which refers to the amount of calories the body needs to digest food. In a healthy individual, the body will burn an extra 10 percent of calories to digest food. But in those who are malnourished, this number can exceed 30 percent by week four of treatment.[3] This physiological response to refeeding requires higher energy requirements and thus more food. It can be difficult, but there is no way around this aspect of your physiology.

Many individuals in recovery wonder how much weight they should be gaining each week. Am I gaining too much? Too slowly? Two to three pounds a week is expected for those in a higher level of care, such as a partial hospitalization program or an intensive outpatient program.[4] The reality of outpatient work might be that any forward progress is positive. If working with a treatment team, it's important they keep a close eye on whether you are making sufficient progress. Studies show that the faster weight gain is accomplished, the better the prognosis.[5]

Could Your ED Be Sabotaging Treatment?

It can be frustrating when you are working hard to eat enough, yet you simply can't keep up with your nutrition goals. If the goal is weight gain, do you really *want* to gain weight? We know many will have mixed feelings about this. You may want to gain weight to get better, but you may also feel scared. Which aspect is dominating your thoughts the most? Sometimes when fear dominates, it can show up in ways that sabotage your efforts. This might look like leaving food behind on your plate, missing a meal/snack or both, or eating in a messy way, spilling food off your plate instead of actually eating it.

Too much movement can also get in the way of success. Are you moving more than you realize? If you walk to a friend's house, walk the dog, or go hiking, don't forget to add more food. These COUNT! You may feel that if you don't sweat, your heart rate isn't elevated, so it doesn't or shouldn't count. That is the ED talking! From a physiological perspective, the body is active and working and will need more food to cover for these different activities. We recommend cutting back on these types of activities if they place too much demand on the body during nutrition rehabilitation.

Behaviors That Might Set You Back in Your Progress

- **Food:** Leaving food behind on the plate, throwing food away or giving it to friends, feeding food to pets, eating in a messy way, not following the meal plan, missing meals or snacks, dissecting food into tiny bites

- **Exercise:** Moving more than you realize, standing instead of sitting, taking the stairs too often, walking instead of driving, shaking your feet or moving instead of sitting still, going on extra walks or doing more exercise but not adding more food

- **Treatment:** Avoiding scheduling with a treatment provider, missing appointments, showing up for sessions but not being present, not doing any of the homework assigned by your providers, not recruiting support people

Baseline Review

We hope that, by now, you've been able to practice using either the 50% or the 33% baseline plates. Before we discuss adding more, let's make sure you have achieved the following plate recommendations.

1. Are you eating 3 meals and 2 snacks per day? If so, it's likely time for a third snack.

2. Are your plates full? Is there any blank space on the plate? Where there's space, there isn't food. Aim for these plates to be entirely full.

3. Are you following the 33% grains/starch plate? If so, try increasing to the 50% grains/starch plate.

4. Have you included a source of dairy (or dairy alternative) with your meals? If not, dairy is an excellent source of calories, proteins, fats, and calcium and would be a great addition to your diet. This

can also be a dairy equivalent, such as pea protein or soy milk or oat milk yogurt.

5.   Are you choosing "safe" or low-fat foods such as plain chicken breast, plain pasta, or steamed veggies? If so, try adding in sauces and fats, and perhaps a few chicken thighs instead of chicken breast. Did you used to love chicken piccata or Parmesan? Go for it! If you are microwaving or steaming vegetables, consider adding fats. This might be scary, but fats add pleasure and taste.

Now Let's Ramp Up to Our Accelerated Plate

If you are already following the previous suggestions, great job! You're ready for this next step. For those with higher energy requirements, this section begins our recommendations for using the Accelerated Plate. This will not be about "weight gain" for everyone, as for many this will be about your specific needs for weight maintenance. Following is a list of ideas to increase the caloric density of meals and snacks. You don't need to make these changes all at once. You might start with one idea, see if it helps meet your goals, then add more strategies as needed. As you add food, your metabolism will increase, which means that to keep up with your metabolism, you will have to add more food over time.

Add juices or an extra glass of milk. Liquid is easily digestible and leaves the stomach quickly, reducing feelings of fullness. Drinks are usually well digested. Try replacing 8 ounces of water with something more nourishing, like 8 ounces (or more) of juice or milk. Some may resist this idea because the ED has avoided juice, thinking it's "unhealthy" or contains "added sugar." But these calories and added sugar will serve to renourish the body. You can add juice or milk first to all meals, then to all snacks, too, substantially increasing your caloric intake by that one change alone. You can also reach for a larger cup or top off your current cup.

Increase your snack size: Snacks can be increased by volume and frequency. If your snack already consists of 2 food groups, increase it to 3. For example, if you are having a yogurt and granola (2-item snack), add some nuts to make it a 3-item snack. If you are having a 3-item snack, increase to 4 (for example, by doubling the quantity of nuts or adding a glass of juice). If you are eating 2 snacks a day, try increasing that to 3. Typically, snacks follow this pattern: Breakfast, Snack (#1), Lunch, Snack (#2), Dinner, Snack (#3). But those who sleep in and stay up late may prefer their schedule to look like this: Breakfast, Lunch, Snack (#1), Dinner, Snack (#2), Snack (#3).

Aim for a "heaping half": In the accelerated rehabilitation phase, it's time to add dimension to your plate. Convert that 50% grains/starches plate to a *heaping* half plate of grains/starches. This heaping half plate should be a mound and not a flat surface. This enables you to increase the volume of grains/starches without altering the proportions of each food group.

Add an extra food group to each meal: You can add an extra food group of your choice to each meal to boost the total volume. If your meals currently contain grains/starches, protein, fruit/vegetables, dairy, and fats, we invite you to choose any food group and add it to your meal. For example, if the meal consists of steak, rice, roasted broccoli (with olive oil), and milk, you can add a buttered dinner roll as the additional food group.

Add an appetizer or dessert or both to all meals: You can also decide to plate a full meal and add an appetizer and/or dessert on the side. This might look like chicken marsala, angel hair pasta with Parmesan cheese, sautéed kale in olive oil, with a few mozzarella sticks or a caprese salad as the appetizer and/or tiramisu as dessert.

Add a ready-to-drink supplement: Adding a supplement such as Ensure Plus, BOOST Plus, Carnation Breakfast Essentials, Orgain, Kate Farms, or any generic version of these can be a quick and easy way to add calories. Because these shakes are nutrient dense and liquid, they are easy to digest and will leave your stomach fairly quickly. You can add as many shakes per day as needed to achieve your nutrition goals! What's nice about an added shake is that they are very easy to remove down the road if your needs change.

Add smoothies or milkshakes: Smoothies are a great way to combine food groups into liquid form, which reduces volume. It's possible, however, to develop an overreliance on shakes and smoothies. We see shakes as a "supplement"—meaning "in addition to" your meal plan, and not a "meal replacement." Some people wonder about adding protein powder to smoothies. This can increase fullness, which is counterproductive for some but may be okay for others. Ingredients that taste good together are generally dairy, dairy alternatives (except for almond milk, which is very low in calories and not helpful in making a calorically dense smoothie), fruit, juice, nut butter, nuts, oats, flaxseeds, and chia seeds. You can also add ice cream or sherbet to increase caloric density.

Use flavored milk instead of plain milk: You can use chocolate, vanilla, strawberry, or other flavored milks. Or you can add Carnation Instant Breakfast powder to milk with meals. Many of the plant-based milk alternatives come flavored as well.

Add more fats
- Add cream-based sauces to pasta, potatoes, and cooked veggies.
- Choose mashed potatoes (made with cream and butter) instead of roasted potatoes.
- Choose twice-baked potato or a loaded potato (with sour cream, butter, and cheese).
- Make "fortified rice"—rice made with coconut milk or mixed with butter.
- Use olive oil when cooking. Only 30 percent is retained in the food, so be sure to add more right before serving.
- Include fried foods like french fries or fried fish.
- Add a source of fat to your sandwiches. Consider avocado, mayo,

butter, nut butter, or hummus. Increase the quantity of these fats in your sandwich.

- Melt cheese on top of your veggies.
- Use whole milk products instead of reduced-fat versions.

Add more calorically dense snacks

- Choose ice cream, cookies, brownies, pie, or pastries for snacks.
- Energy bites add more density without a lot of volume.
- Granola bars, trail mix, or nuts can be helpful.

CHAPTER 7

Putting It All Together: Meal and Snack Ideas

THIS CHAPTER IS dedicated to putting the plate together and making sure you have an idea of "what is enough." You'll find examples of meals and snacks so that you have a better idea of what yours can look like. Throughout this chapter, we'll help you learn how to assess your meals to ensure they are adequate using the Plate-by-Plate Approach® and discuss ways each plate can be improved.

PLATE-BY-PLATE: BREAKFAST

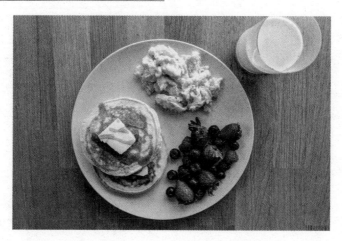

Food Group Checklist

Grains/starches—2 pancakes with syrup

Protein—scrambled eggs

Vegetables or fruit—berries

Fat—butter (on pancakes)

Dairy or dairy alternative—milk

Final Review Questions

Are all food groups present? Grains/starches? Protein? Fruits/veggies? Dairy? Fat? Yes!

Is the plate 50% grains/starches? Is it 25% protein? Is it 25% fruit or veggies? Does it have dairy and fats? Yes! It looks like 33% starch, but if you placed those pancakes next to each other it would fill half of the plate with grains/starches.

Is the whole plate full? No. There's a little room left on the plate. For some, this meal is adequate, but others might require more. For example, if you're in need of weight gain, if you have higher energy requirements, if your vital signs are unstable, or if you are finding you feel hungry or are bingeing after this meal, you might need to add more.

Does the meal "make sense" and feel cohesive? Yes!

Have you challenged your ED? Yes! This breakfast may challenge the ED for many. If it doesn't, what else can you have for breakfast that will challenge it?

Recommendation

- Closely consider your needs. If more food is needed, try increasing the portion of eggs or fruit on the plate or increase to the Accelerated Plate.

PLATE-BY-PLATE: LUNCH

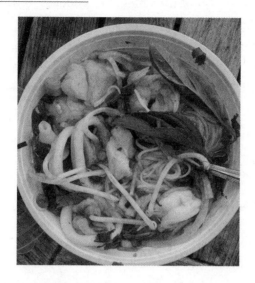

Food Group Checklist

Grains/starches—noodles

Protein—mixed seafood

Vegetables or fruit—mung bean sprouts, green onion, basil

Fat—very little in the broth

Dairy—none

Final Review Questions

Are all food groups present? Grains/starches? Protein? Fruits/veggies? Dairy? Fat? No. This meal is missing fat and dairy.

Is the plate 50% grains/starches? Is it 25% protein? Is it 25% fruit or veggies? Does it have dairy and fats? No. This meal is served in a bowl, and while that can make it tricky to determine how much of each food group is present, we have a few tips. First, make sure your meal is served in a large bowl versus a cup. Take note of what food groups are present in that bowl. Then imagine you poured it on a 10-inch dinner plate. Would it fill the plate? Are there enough noodles in there to fill half the plate?

A typical bowl of pho contains adequate noodles to fulfill the grains/starches category. If it's easier, you can always plate up the different food groups before combining with broth to ensure adequate portions.

Is the whole plate full? No. This bowl is missing fat and dairy.

Does the meal "make sense" and feel cohesive? Yes!

Have you challenged your ED? Yes!

Recommendations

- Add an egg roll for fat.
- Add a Vietnamese coffee (made with sweetened condensed milk) for dairy.

PLATE-BY-PLATE: DINNER

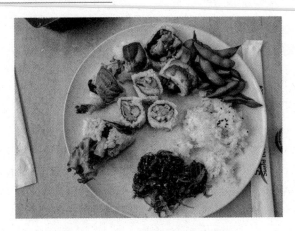

Food Group Checklist

Grains/starches—rice (in sushi roll and on plate)

Protein—tempura shrimp (in sushi roll), edamame

Vegetables or fruit—seaweed salad, lettuce/cucumber (in sushi roll)

Fat—avocado (in sushi roll)

Dairy—none

Final Review Questions

Are all food groups present? Grains/starches? Protein? Fruits/veggies? Dairy? Fat? No. This meal is missing dairy. For some cuisines, it doesn't make sense to add dairy, or dairy isn't available with the meal. For this meal, consider adding more of something else in its place. Perhaps adding a few more pieces of sushi or a beverage like sweetened iced tea (this won't replace the nutritional content of milk but it will increase the total volume of the plate to help meet your needs).

Is the plate 50% grains/starches? Is it 25% protein? Is it 25% fruit or veggies? Does it have dairy and fats? No, there is some rice around the sushi roll but not enough to fill the equivalent of half the plate. The extra rice plated on the side helps fill that requirement. The protein in this meal is similar. There's some in the sushi roll but not quite enough to equal 25% of the plate. The edamame beans add protein to this meal. There is avocado for fats, but no dairy present.

Is the whole plate full? No. There's still room left on the plate. For some, this meal is adequate; for others who will need more, try filling it up a bit more (add more rice, sushi, or edamame).

Does the meal "make sense" and feel cohesive? Yes!

Have you challenged your ED? Yes!

Recommendations

- Add something else to cover for the missing dairy: extra sushi or a sweetened iced tea. While this wouldn't provide added calcium, it would help with added volume.
- Closely consider your needs. If more food is needed, increase the portion of rice, sushi, or edamame or move to the Accelerated Plate.

PLATE-BY-PLATE: ACCELERATED PLATE

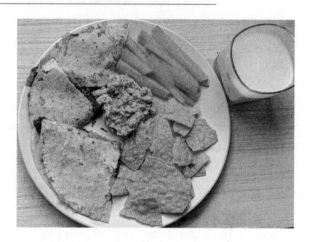

Food Group Checklist

Grains/starches—tortilla, chips

Protein—beans (in quesadilla)

Vegetables or fruit—carrot sticks

Fat—guacamole

Dairy—cheese (in quesadilla), milk

Final Review Questions

Are all food groups present? Grains/starches? Protein? Fruits/veggies? Dairy? Fat? Yes!

Is the plate 50% grains/starches? Is it 25% protein? Is it 25% fruit or veggies? Does it have dairy and fats? Yes!

Is the whole plate full? Yes!

Does the meal "make sense" and feel cohesive? Yes!

Have you challenged your ED? Yes!

Recommendations

- Consider your needs. If more food is needed, add more guacamole or melt some additional cheese on the chips for a side of nachos, consider adding sour cream, or increase the volume of milk. If that feels like too much at this meal, consider other meals/snacks you can add to for increased volume.

PLATE-BY-PLATE: VEGAN PLATE

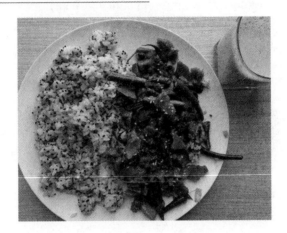

Food Group Checklist

Grains/starches—rice/quinoa

Protein—apricot seitan (plant-based protein made of wheat gluten)

Vegetables or fruit—green beans (in seitan)

Fat—none (other than a little bit of oil used to sauté the seitan and veggies)

Dairy alternative—soy milk

Final Review Questions

Are all food groups present? Grains/starches? Protein? Fruits/veggies? Dairy? Fat? No. There is very little fat present in this meal, other than what was used to sauté the seitan and veggies. Try adding cashews to the seitan and veggie mixture or add vegan butter to the rice/quinoa mixture after cooking.

Is the plate 50% grains/starches? Is it 25% protein? Is it 25% fruit or veggies? Does it have dairy and fats? Yes! The seitan/veggie mixture fills half the plate but is fairly evenly divided between both food groups.

Is the whole plate full? Yes, although depending on your needs, there's a bit of room on the edge of the plate to increase volume.

Does the meal "make sense" and feel cohesive? Yes!

Have you challenged your ED? Yes!

Recommendations

- Add fat to this meal. The amount of oil used to sauté the seitan/veggie mixture may not be adequate. Consider adding cashews to the seitan/veggie mixture or vegan butter to the rice/quinoa mixture after cooking.

- If this volume of food is inadequate to meet your needs, consider filling up the plate a bit more.

PLATE-BY-PLATE: SNACKS

Snacks are recommended for everyone. They help regulate blood sugar and energy levels throughout the day, fill in nutritional gaps, and increase the quantity of food consumed while helping to keep the volume of food at meals more manageable. They're also a great way to practice food exposure! You might plan to visit a café with a friend or buy a few new (and fun!) snack items at the grocery store (see chapter 16 for more information on this important recovery skill).

We recommend you start with 2 snacks each day that include 2 items each. An "item" refers to a food item from one of the 5 food groups and is equal to a typical serving of that food. For example, one serving of nuts or one serving of crackers. Using a smaller side plate (~6 inches in diameter), add crackers to half the plate. That would be considered 1 "item." Fill the other half of that plate with sliced cheese. That's your second "item." As your individual nutrition needs change, you may need more than two 2-item snacks. See examples of 2-, 3-, and 4-item snacks below.

**2-ITEM SNACK:
PAN DULCE + LATTE**

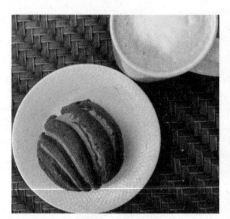

**3-ITEM SNACK:
APPLE SLICES, CHEESE,
MIXED NUTS**

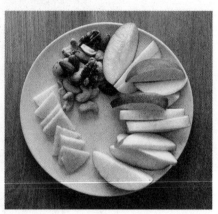

**2-ITEM SNACK:
SAVORY CRACKER MIX +
PERSIMMON**

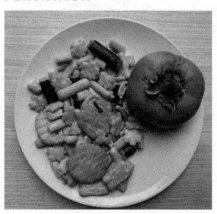

**3-ITEM SNACK:
CHOCOLATE CAKE,
RASPBERRIES, MILK**

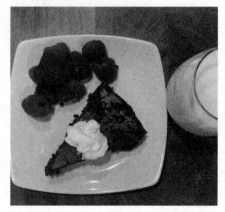

4-ITEM SNACK: CRACKERS, CHEESE, SALAMI, GRAPES

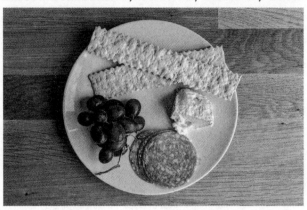

4-ITEM SNACK: CRACKERS, HUMMUS, APPLE, SWEETENED ICED TEA

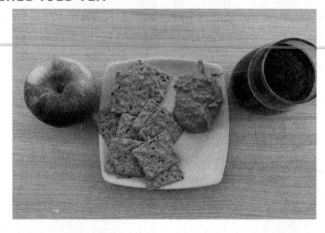

CHAPTER 8

An Approach for All

THE **PLATE-BY-PLATE APPROACH**® was developed for use by anyone with an ED, no matter the diagnosis. With an emphasis on plating meals and snacks visually, and a structure of 3 meals and at least 2 snacks per day, the approach can be applied for many who are struggling to nourish themselves through an ED. Throughout this chapter, we will show you how this approach can be used in the nutritional management of BED, anorexia nervosa, avoidant/restrictive food intake disorder, and bulimia nervosa.

Binge Eating Disorder (BED)

A primary cause of binge eating is food restriction. In fact, BED is typically characterized by periods of restriction followed by periods of bingeing. This usually results in increased feelings of guilt, shame, and depression, leading back to restriction. This cycle maintains the binge behavior. For those struggling with BED, the Plate-by-Plate Approach® provides structure and consistency to eating in order to regulate blood sugar and hormones associated with hunger and satiety and to ensure balanced nutrition to help reduce binge episodes.

BED can occur in people of all sizes, though it is mistakenly thought to occur only in people in larger bodies. For those in smaller bodies, BED can be missed by providers or not taken seriously. For those with BED in larger bodies, providers mistakenly prescribe "weight loss," which perpetuates the restrictive cycle. It's critical to understand that bigger bodies need *more* food, not less. If your nutrition is inadequate, cravings will increase, and you will be more vulnerable to emotional triggers to binge (stress, shifts in mood, and boredom). The physiological drive for food in a deprived state is powerful, and the body will be more likely to seek out food in an uncontrolled way. Establishing the right amount of food to nourish the body to prevent binges will allow those with BED to stabilize eating behaviors so that the body can relax and truly be fed.

Case Example: Luis

Luis is a thirty-five-year-old man with BED. He has lived in a larger body his entire life and describes himself as a "chronic dieter." As a child, he was frequently put on diets by his doctors and his parents, never once feeling able to lose weight. As a result of dieting, he remembers "sneaking" food late at night after his parents went to bed. He would grab anything he could find, especially foods his doctors and parents told him to avoid (chips, soda, candy, and cookies). He always felt out of control around these foods as a kid, and even as an adult he would avoid buying them because he didn't "trust himself" not to binge on them. Luis finally got so fed up with the constant restrict/binge cycle that he sought help from an RD using the Plate-by-Plate Approach®.

He was instructed to eat 3 meals following the 50% plate and 3 snacks per day (2 items per snack). There was even the recommendation to include some of the foods Luis had been told to avoid, gradually, such as chips at lunch. Luis felt like it was "too much food" and was worried it would lead to further weight gain. Initially, Luis ate only 2 meals and 2 snacks each day, restricting breakfast and morning snack, thinking that would be helpful to prevent weight gain. He thought that, since his binge eating occurred mostly in the afternoon/evening, maybe by eating more during that time, he would avoid the binges while still restricting overall intake to prevent weight gain.

Luis was surprised to find that he was still bingeing, despite eating consistently in the afternoon, and as a result, he continued to gain weight. He felt terrible about the binge episodes. Luis finally told his dietitian what was going on and committed to eating all 3 meals and snacks each day. It seemed like so much food; he was so used to dieting, counting calories, and eating less. His dietitian assured him eating regularly would help to prevent binge eating. Luis was still apprehensive about including in those meals and snacks the foods he commonly binged on, but agreed to add them in gradually. After a few months of eating 3 meals and 3 snacks per day, Luis went from bingeing twice each day to less than once per week. He felt better, both emotionally and physically, and to his surprise, his weight stabilized because he was bingeing so much less. He noticed he felt increasingly confident eating the foods he previously binged on. He was able to have chips and a soda with a sandwich at lunch without feeling out of control. He would have Oreo cookies with a glass of milk as an afternoon snack and felt satisfied with a few cookies, no longer reaching for the entire bag. Luis still felt the desire to lose weight, but agreed to work on his body image with his therapist while continuing to practice eating consistent and adequate meals and snacks each day.

Like Luis, those with BED will need to eat 3 meals and 2 or 3 snacks per day to obtain enough nutrition to meet the body's needs and prevent binges. Consistency is important here. Bingeing can occur even if you have had 3 meals and 2 or 3 snacks according to your meal plan, *if the previous day's intake was insufficient.* Skipping meals or snacks without making up for what was missed can result in binge episodes or can increase the vulnerability to bingeing. The body is smart and will seek out food if there is a negative energy imbalance. Cravings will increase, aromas will become more intense, interest in food will heighten, and your overall pull toward food will intensify. Those with high-energy demands, like athletes or those who work on their feet all day, might be more triggered to binge on higher-intensity days (or on days off when they can finally feel their hunger more) if a state of energy imbalance ensues. Using food logs can be helpful in finding these nutritional gaps throughout the week.

Additionally, incorporating into meals and snacks those foods that you are most likely to binge on helps neutralize any power they hold and allows you to practice eating them in quantities that feel manageable.

Anorexia Nervosa (AN)

Those with anorexia nervosa will have elevated metabolic needs in order to gain weight while repairing any systems that have been compromised by severe food restriction. It's common in anorexia for caloric needs to rise sharply during the early stages of refeeding. To initiate and keep up with this metabolic recovery, we recommend that those with AN follow the 50% plate to start at 3 meals and include 3 snacks per day (2 items per snack). Those with AN binge/purge type might need to initially start out with the 33% plate (33% grains/starch), until binge/purge behaviors are reduced. The 33% plate might enable those with AN binge/purge type to increase volume while practicing keeping the food down. They can then progress to the 50% plate to work on weight restoration.

We also encourage those with AN to include feared foods from the start. This exposure to feared foods will help reduce anxiety around these foods over time. Once consistently eating 3 meals (50% plate) and 3 snacks (2 items each) per day, those with AN will likely need to increase what they are eating to promote continued weight gain and metabolic recovery. The Accelerated Plate is often appropriate at this stage to help individuals with AN meet their nutritional goals when the body becomes hypermetabolic and weight gain becomes more "calorically expensive." For more on how to achieve this, see chapter 6.

Case Study: Aiko

Aiko is a twenty-three-year-old nonbinary biological female with anorexia nervosa. Aiko just graduated from college and is living alone for the first time while navigating a new job. They struggled with restrictive eating and weight loss during college but never received a formal ED diagnosis or treatment. Aiko has not had a period since they were 20 years old and is approximately twenty pounds lighter than their previous high weight. They are often fatigued, chronically cold, dizzy upon standing, and they think about food constantly.

When Aiko goes to see a new primary care physician to establish care, they are diagnosed with AN and referred to an RD who uses the Plate-by-Plate Approach®. The dietitian recommends that Aiko begin including more variety at meals, besides just oatmeal at breakfast and rice at lunch and dinner.

Aiko is a competent cook but is terrified to increase what they are eating. The thought of adding in different foods makes them extremely anxious. The team Aiko is working with strongly encourages them to take a medical leave from their job and return home to live with their parents while undergoing treatment. Determined to maintain their independence and motivated by their new job, Aiko makes the tough decision to stay where they are while undergoing treatment. Aiko's team decides to give them a trial run of outpatient treatment while living on their own and sets them up on the Recovery Record app for meal plan accountability, which Aiko uses to log photos of meals and snacks that their team can see. Aiko commits to eating 3 meals and 3 snacks per day, to have weekly weight and vital sign checks, as well as weekly check-ins with their RD and therapist. Aiko's physician recommends that Aiko stop all exercise activity "for now" until the resolution of their bradycardia (which is defined as a heart rate less than 60 beats per minute) and orthostasis (change of 20 beats per minute in pulse or blood pressure when changing from reclining to standing position).

As Aiko begins eating more food, they experience increased fullness, constipation, and bloating. This makes it hard to adhere completely to the recommendations from the dietitian, but nevertheless, they make progress. As treatment continues and they need more food, they struggle with volume. Aiko's dietitian suggests using liquid nutrition for part of the meal. They also educate Aiko about how to reduce the volume of vegetables on the plate to minimize digestive discomfort associated with eating too much fiber. Lastly, the dietitian encourages Aiko to make foods more calorically dense and to choose calorically dense snacks. Aiko continued to struggle with the fear of weight gain but remained motivated by their independence and were able to incorporate many of these suggestions to promote medical stability.

As the weeks passed, Aiko became more comfortable with the dietary and exercise changes. They started gaining consistent weight, their vital signs improved, and the initial digestive symptoms they experienced (fullness, constipation, bloating) resolved. Eventually, Aiko was cleared by their physician to incorporate light activity again (walking, yoga). Aiko leaned on a couple of close friends they made in their apartment complex for meal accountability, making regular lunch and dinner dates with them. Aiko also shared their diagnosis and treatment goals with their family, who began to visit more often to check in. Aiko, now close to weight-restored, still hasn't seen their period return. However, their physician is confident that it will return within one to two months, as long as they get to, and stay in, their goal-weight range. Aiko continues to work on incorporating feared foods into their diet but has become more confident with many of the foods they used to fear most.

To gain weight and resolve vital signs and hormonal abnormalities, those like Aiko with AN will need to eat more food than they are likely comfortable with. This can be challenging to do alone, and many require support from friends and family to maintain motivation for recovery. What starts out as 3 meals and 3 snacks per day following the 50% plate may quickly increase to the Accelerated Plate, relying on calorically dense meals and snacks plus shakes to meet needs. It can feel as if you are constantly "chasing" your metabolism during this phase of treatment with no end in sight. However, with some creative planning with your RD, as well as finding internal and external motivation, this process can be successful.

Avoidant/Restrictive Food Intake Disorder

Patients with avoidant/restrictive food intake disorder, or ARFID, may experience malnutrition and make narrow food choices due to any or all of the following.

1. Fear of the consequences that eating may have on their body (pain, vomiting)

2. Sensory sensitivities (food feels too "slimy," "cold," or "mushy," for example)

3. A general lack of interest in eating, with few hunger cues

This leads to weight loss, bradycardia and orthostasis, compromised growth (children/adolescents), reduced bone density, and multiple vitamin and mineral deficiencies as a result of their limited food choices. There is often not a concern for body image or weight (as in AN), and patients may even report wanting to gain weight (unlike AN). An individual with ARFID can also be at a weight that is normal for their body, but they may have multiple vitamin and mineral deficiencies due to lack of variety in their diet. ARFID can be effectively treated through intensive exposure work, desensitizing the individual to feared foods in a hierarchical format.

Utilizing the Plate-by-Plate Approach®, an individual with ARFID can learn how to fill their plate with adequate volume and variety by incorporating foods they are comfortable with in each food group and gradually practicing exposure to new or challenging foods. Over time, their diet becomes more varied, correcting any underlying nutritional deficiencies and medical instabilities.

Case Study: Max

Max is a forty-year-old man with a lifelong history of limited food preferences, as well as chronic constipation without any known cause. When Max was seven years old, he choked on a hot dog at a baseball game. Max's parents made an unsuccessful attempt at the Heimlich maneuver, after which EMTs had to manually remove the hot dog from his esophagus. Fortunately, Max survived this horrific incident, but his relationship with food after that was forever altered.

As time went on, the list of foods Max was willing to eat narrowed. He initially avoided all round foods that felt like choking hazards (carrots, hot dogs, sausages, grapes, hard candies), which progressed to avoiding all hard/crunchy foods (raw/crunchy fruits and veggies, crunchy chips, toast), and eventually all meat. Max was limited to a soft/puréed diet of mostly white foods (white rice, soft white bread, mashed potatoes, macaroni and white cheddar cheese, milk, yogurt). He feared anything that could potentially get "stuck" in his esophagus, and his anxiety was so extreme around these foods that he couldn't tolerate eating with others (for fear they would choke as well).

Throughout his life, Max was thought to be a "really picky eater." At every well-child check growing up, his parents were told, "He'll grow out of it" and "Keep offering new foods, and he'll try them eventually." But Max never did. Throughout adolescence, his weight and height slowed down prematurely. Max is now still significantly underweight and never reached his maximum potential height. As Max got older, he couldn't eat with others and was so anxious about eating away from his house that he avoided these situations at all costs. The isolation caused depression.

During a routine medical exam, Max spoke with his physician about his struggles with food and constipation. The physician was savvy about EDs and diagnosed him with ARFID, as well as gastroparesis (slowed gut motility from chronic malnutrition and lack of dietary fiber). His doctor referred him to a team of specialists to help him recover. Max was both relieved to finally have an answer and nervous about treatment. When Max met with his RD, his diet was assessed.

Assessment of Max's Diet

Breakfast—1 bowl of vanilla yogurt, 1 bowl of applesauce, 1 glass of 2% milk

Lunch—1 bowl of mac and cheese, 1 bowl of applesauce

Snack—2 pieces of soft white bread with butter, 1 glass of 2% milk

Dinner—1 bowl of white rice with butter, 1 piece of soft white buttered bread, 1 glass of apple juice

Snack—1 bowl of mashed potatoes with butter, 1 glass of 2% milk

Max's diet was sufficient in fat as well as calcium and vitamin D but lacking in overall calories, protein, fiber, iron, vitamin B12, as well other vitamins and minerals. The dietitian worked with Max to use the Plate-by-Plate Approach® to help him boost his energy, protein, and nutritional needs to support weight restoration while using his current list of acceptable foods for his meals and snacks. Max was encouraged to switch to a 10-inch dish to make sure he was plating enough. At breakfast, Max was typically getting 3 of 5 food groups. He was able to add an additional cup of milk (for added protein) and 2 pieces of white bread (grains) with butter (fats). He was able to rotate in cereal with milk for added iron, B12, and fiber, as well as oatmeal.

At lunch, he was typically getting 3 of 5 food groups. Max was able to add vanilla yogurt (dairy) and a glass of apple juice (fruit) to fill the plate and balance the meal. At dinner, where he would normally have 3 of 5 food groups, he was able to add a tall glass of milk (1 serving is the dairy, 1 serving is protein) and a morning snack to help increase the volume of food.

Max agreed to take a multivitamin to make sure he was getting enough vitamins and minerals until his diet could be fully expanded. He also agreed to work on some exposure, after the dietitian talked about how the process might go. He said he would be willing to try pasta with melted cheese on it, which was a slight pivot from the mac and cheese he was eating daily. He also expressed interest in trying cheese tortellini and ravioli. He would cook them, the dietitian explained, and have just a few bites as a side to his entrée. Max was asked to track how often he had these new foods. His dietitian reminded him that it could take fifteen to twenty times before he might "like" the food. Increased comfort wouldn't come until Max had tried each food many times.

Max was relieved that his dietitian gave him ways to increase his volume of food using his "safe" foods rather than incorporating a bunch of new foods that he was too anxious to eat. He was excited because all the suggestions felt so doable!

He was able to incorporate a wider variety of protein sources, fruits, and vegetables, and is beginning to try new textures of food. He will continue this exposure work with his dietitian to increase his repertoire of acceptable foods. Through this journey, he has also been working with his therapist to reduce anxiety when eating with others. Max has been able to eat with his family and close friends more often and is beginning to feel less anxious and more social.

Like Max, individuals struggling with ARFID may have limited ability to eat outside their own house. It can be anxiety-provoking and even debilitating to eat when a food is unknown. Work on exposure is key to building confidence in eating and reducing anxiety around food for those with ARFID. The Plate-by-Plate Approach® is a gentle way to show those with ARFID how to turn their small list of preferred foods into full plates that are balanced (if lacking in cohesion) and adequate. These advancements improve nutritional deficiencies, help meet such medical goals as improving vital signs, weight restoration, hormonal balance, metabolic recovery, mood, and energy level. This approach also allows individuals with ARFID to build confidence in eating as they expand their palate.

Bulimia Nervosa (BN)

An individual struggling with bulimia nervosa may experience bouts of food restriction, followed by binge eating, then compensatory behaviors (purging, diet pill or laxative abuse, or exercise). Medical complications of BN may include those common to AN, and additionally electrolyte abnormalities (low potassium, sodium, phosphorus, and magnesium, for example). These are typically corrected with adequate nutritional intake and cessation of compensatory behaviors.

Those with BN often struggle with food volume, especially in the case of purging and laxative abuse. The feeling of having food in the stomach or intestines can be very uncomfortable, so food volume should always be taken into consideration. The Plate-by-Plate Approach® can be especially helpful to those struggling with BN, as there are a variety of ways to construct the plate to support one's recovery needs. Using the 33% plate is generally a first step. Working with a registered dietitian to determine your needs will help an individual with BN start out with a lower-volume plate without sacrificing adequate nutrition and encourage the confidence to build to and tolerate a higher volume of food.

Case Study: Nidhi

Nidhi is a sixty-five-year-old woman with bulimia nervosa (BN). Nidhi's
BN behaviors began later in life, after she hit menopause and became
increasingly dissatisfied with her midsection. She was newly widowed, lonely,
depressed, and her bingeing and purging took her by surprise. Nidhi knew
this wasn't a healthy behavior, but she felt desperate to lose the weight
gained through menopause. She finally started dating again, slowly, and
was more self-conscious about her older body. Over time, Nidhi engaged in
other compensatory behaviors as well, including laxative and diet pill use, and
walking miles each day to "burn off the calories" from binge episodes and even
regular meals. She felt out of control.

At a dental visit, Nidhi's dentist noticed she had erosion of her enamel
and more cavities than at previous visits. The dentist asked about her eating
habits as well as her dental hygiene, and Nidhi decided to be honest. She
told her dentist about the binge eating and purging. This was the first person
she had ever confided in, and she was nervous to hear her dentist's response.
Fortunately, her dentist was very understanding and compassionate. Nidhi's
dentist encouraged her to reach out to her primary doctor for a thorough
workup and directed Nidhi to the website for NEDA (National Eating
Disorders Association) to get further information about and support. Nidhi
was grateful for the information and scheduled a visit with her primary doctor.

At that visit, her doctor made the BN diagnosis and referred her to an RD
for further nutrition counseling. Nidhi met with the RD, motivated to end the
cycle of restrict/binge/purge. She wanted to get her life back, to start living
again.

The RD educated Nidhi about the importance of meeting baseline
nutrition needs to prevent bingeing and purging, and he explained that any
food restriction would lead to bingeing and purging. The only way to reduce
these behaviors is to eat regular, balanced, and adequate meals and snacks
throughout the day. It was recommended that Nidhi start with the 33%
plate at meals and eat 2 snacks per day, including 2 food items. She was also
encouraged to dispose of all diet pills and laxatives.

Nidhi tried to use distraction techniques, such as volunteering locally and
painting when she felt the urge to purge. The first week was incredibly hard.

Nidhi experienced many urges to purge and was in intense pain at the end of each day, due to slowed gut motility after years of laxative abuse. She spoke to her doctor, who recommended hot packs, drinking warm beverages, and light walking. The doctor told Nidhi that it would take time for her body to adjust to the feeling of keeping food down and allowing it to move through the digestive tract normally. She implemented the tips her doctor provided for slowed gut motility. She had more energy. She didn't get tired as much. But she was very uncomfortable with her body. She stuck with 3 meals and 2 snacks per day, though it was often hard to do on days when she was feeling down. But she knew that if she skipped a meal, she would be more likely to binge and purge. Slowly, she began to realize that a week would go by without an episode, then it was 10 days, then a month! It took time, but her body began to run normally again and Nidhi was able to build confidence eating adequate and higher-volume meals.

Like Nidhi, those with bulimia nervosa will struggle most with consistency and structure of eating, volume of food, and urges to purge or otherwise compensate for eating. Working with an RD to implement 3 balanced and adequate meals (while ensuring that you are consuming enough volume) and 2 to 3 snacks per day will help keep your metabolism stimulated throughout the day, regulate blood sugar levels, keep energy levels up, and minimize the triggers for bingeing and purging.

Reducing, and eventually eliminating, all compensatory behaviors takes persistence and time, but the longer you stick to a structured eating plan and the longer you go between compensatory episodes, the easier it will become. As you cut back on compensatory behaviors like purging and laxative use, be sure to check with a medical doctor to assess your lab work. You may also wish to discuss alternative strategies for maintaining bowel health to help prevent constipation.

Anxiety and distress levels can be high when you are trying to eliminate compensatory mechanisms. Incorporating distraction after eating can be helpful to get through the time period immediately following meals. These include watching a favorite show, reading a book, meditation, calling a friend, gentle yoga, playing with your dog, or enlisting a friend or loved one to sit with you after meals to ensure you don't purge.

There are many ways the Plate-by-Plate Approach® can be helpful for BED, anorexia nervosa, ARFID, and bulimia nervosa. This no-numbers, no-counting approach allows a person to eat with regularity and consistency, while consuming an amount that is "enough." This helps to reduce the vulnerability to binge, purge, or use laxatives, which can happen after a period of caloric restriction. Across time, this allows you to meet your medical goals—improved vital signs, weight, metabolism, hormones, mood, and energy. It's not easy to eat more and include foods that your ED has deemed to be "off-limits." But if your current way hasn't been working for you, perhaps you might want to try something new? You've got this!

CHAPTER 9

Barriers to Following the Plate-by-Plate Approach®

SO YOU'VE EMBARKED on your recovery journey, you're doing your part to get better, and now you feel awful! What the heck?! No one said this would be easy. It can't be. If it were easy, everyone with an ED would be fully recovered. This is hard.

But you know what? Your effort will be worth it. While there might not be a quick fix, and while the path might be bumpy, you are on your way to a more peaceful relationship with food, movement, and your body. This chapter will provide you with tools to ease any pain you're feeling throughout this process.

If you've been restricting your food intake, bingeing, purging, using diet pills or laxatives, or overexercising, your body's health is compromised. Learning to eat enough, keep food down, balance your plates, and find consistency and adequacy in your diet will help you restore health but will initially feel uncomfortable. Many people experience physical symptoms, including constipation, bloating, and nausea, and psychological barriers like a reduced or increased appetite due to stress, anxiety, and depression, when they first begin to follow the Plate-by-Plate Approach®. Some are socially isolated or lack financial resources for treatment or the motivation to continue. We want you to know that these situations are common and normal. In this chapter we will explore strategies for coping with these concerns to help you best navigate through recovery.

Gastrointestinal Problems

Common gastrointestinal issues include bloating, gastroparesis (delayed gastric emptying), nausea, constipation, and heartburn (see chapter 11). We will cover some strategies to alleviate these problems, but should they persist, consult with a medical doctor who can assess whether a referral to a gastrointestinal specialist is necessary. A physician may also be able to provide you reassurance that your symptoms are common and expected side effects of ED recovery and not something else. That alone can be immensely reassuring. A doctor may also be able to prescribe medications or other treatments to help ease discomfort.

Watch out for any unintentional vomiting, blood or mucus in your stool, or symptoms that are prolonged and not progressing. These should be immediately checked by a medical doctor, who can decide the best next steps. Sometimes stool testing and further scopes are needed to make diagnostic assessments.

Bloating and Gastroparesis (Delayed Gastric Emptying)

Bloating is very common among individuals who are working through metabolic recovery and nutritional rehabilitation. We see this occur across all diagnoses. Someone with BED might feel bloated as they are trying to eat more regularly throughout the day (a new and maybe uncomfortable feeling). Someone with AN who needs to gain weight might feel bloated as they adjust to the higher-volume meal plan. Someone with BN may feel bloated and struggle with edema as they work on stopping binge/purge behaviors and their body experiences a shift in fluid status. And someone with ARFID may feel bloated if they are constipated because of a limited diet or as they're adjusting to a new meal plan.

Bloating, or abdominal distention, occurs in part because of the delay in gastric emptying (known as "gastroparesis") that results from malnutrition. In other words, the ED has caused a slowdown of your entire system. Normally, food goes into your stomach and is digested.

The stomach may protrude slightly after meals. However, with malnutrition, the food will sit in your stomach, causing you to feel full and bloated for longer periods of time. In those who have been dieting, or eating irregularly or inconsistently, bloating can be more severe and intense, which can add to body image distress. This is not fun for those already struggling in this area. Constipation is also a known cause of bloating and distention (we go into detail below).

One strategy to help with bloating is to work on increasing metabolic recovery through regular and consistent fueling for several consecutive days.[1] The pathway out is through. In our experience, it can take approximately 4 to 5 days before you will notice some improvement. But you will need to be consistent with your changes. Often people must endure some amount of discomfort to recalibrate their metabolism. This will allow you to feel more awake, active, and energetic.

You won't feel hungry during this time. If you listened to hunger during this time, you would be listening to a suppressed metabolism's hunger cues. Pushing forward will lead to metabolic recovery.[2]

Tips

- Smaller meals (the 33% plate) and more frequent snacks (3 snacks) might be helpful here.

- Consider adding liquids like milk, juice, or shakes (Ensure, BOOST, Kate Farms) to help increase calories without adding a lot of volume.

- Avoid high-fiber foods, which can take longer to digest and increase feelings of fullness.

Nausea

Nausea can be caused by many factors: medication side effects, feelings associated with eating more than you are used to, suppressed digestive enzymes, depression, anxiety, stress, allergies, gastrointestinal concerns (constipation, acid reflux, SIBO—small intestinal bacterial overgrowth), abdominal wall dysfunction, pelvic floor dysfunction, inflammatory bowel disease, ulcers, irritable bowel syndrome, dehydration, aversions to smells/textures, trauma, and more.

Many describe a constant, nagging, never-ending nausea. This can be incredibly hard to navigate. We have several tips to help approach your meals while experiencing nausea, because even if you are nauseous, you still need to eat. Skipping meals, missing meals, and/or being at a low weight can exacerbate medical complications associated with malnutrition. It can also reduce the efficacy of any psychotropic medications you might be taking,[3] especially if you are missing out on key nutrients like omega-3 fatty acids, vitamin D, and zinc, which can help improve their effectiveness.[4] Below are some remedies that might be helpful in reducing the feeling of nausea.

Ginger[5]

- Ginger chews or candies can be soothing.
- Ginger capsules contain a higher dose of ginger but are not regulated, so exact dose per pill is unknown. May also help with gastric emptying.[6]
- Ginger tea can be soothing but is known to be a bit weaker.

Peppermint[7]

- Hard candy
- Peppermint essential oils (aromatherapy)
- Extract (may contain ethanol for those needing to avoid alcohol)

OTC

- Iberogast, which contains trace ethanol, can help with nausea and bloating due to IBS (made with nine herbs; available online or in pharmacies)[8]

Alternative techniques

- Distraction
- Breathing exercises
- Stretching/yoga
- Mindfulness

- Guided imagery
- Biofeedback
- Acupuncture/acupressure
- Sea-Bands

Prescription meds

If nausea persists, talk to your medical provider about prescription medications such as ondansetron, hydroxyzine, famotidine, omeprazole, or metoclopramide.

Other considerations

- Hydrate regularly.
- Keep bowels moving regularly.
- Pay attention to times of day when the nausea is worse. For many the morning can be tough. Plan to increase food when nausea subsides!
- Are certain textures or food consistencies better than others?
- Use scents of lemon, lavender, and mint at the table when feeling nauseous; essential oils can really help!
- Enlist family support.
- Of course, consult a doctor.

Constipation

Constipation is a common side effect of weight loss, dieting, malnutrition, and laxative abuse. It can also occur during the refeeding phase. When there is insufficient nutrition, there is usually not enough energy or volume to support digestion and to push food through the digestive tract; in addition, the lack of fats, fiber, and variety fail to keep the gut moving. As you add more food, or change your eating patterns, there can be a backup in digestion and excretion until the metabolism increases enough to normalize the process. Constipation adds to bloating and fullness, making it difficult to feel hungry or to want to eat. This can exacerbate a negative body image.

Working with a medical doctor and considering some of our tips below will be important to help ease this discomfort. Keeping bowels moving regularly will allow you to be more successful with your meal plan. *Stimulant laxatives are not recommended and can cause painful cramping and damage to colonic nerve cells in the long term.*[9]

Tips for Alleviating Constipation

Fiber	**Does your diet contain enough fiber?**
	There are two forms of fiber: insoluble fiber (found in vegetables, whole grain products like breads, crackers, and cereals) and soluble fiber (found in fruits, dried fruit, and oatmeal). Both forms are an important part of the diet. Insoluble fiber bulks up the stools and soluble fiber keeps the stools soft. If your stool is hard, you might require more soluble fiber. If you are not producing much stool, you might need more insoluble fiber.
	Too much fiber can increase bloating and constipation and reduce vitamin and mineral absorption.
Fluids	**Are you hydrating sufficiently?**
	Dehydration can cause dry stools, plus fiber needs fluids to move through the colon. To assess whether you are hydrating enough, look at the color of your urine. Hydrated urine should be pale yellow. Dehydrated urine often resembles apple juice in color.
Fats	**Are you consuming enough fats?**
	Fats should be present with each meal and snack. It helps the stool move through the colon. Without enough dietary fat, the stool will be dry and difficult to pass through the colon.
Overall Volume	**Are you eating enough and at regular intervals?**
	Eating regularly throughout the day, and in an amount that meets your needs, will keep your digestion moving along. Skipping meals can cause a metabolic and digestive slowdown that can increase bloating and constipation.

"I am always full"

We expect that as you aim to increase/regulate your food intake, you are likely to feel full as your body adjusts to eating regularly. The fullness will not last forever. This feeling will dissipate as your metabolism increases. We often say that if the process of getting used to eating more regularly feels "too easy," perhaps you aren't pushing yourself enough (or else maybe your body just responded quickly). Change will take some adjustment.

Tips

1. Distract yourself! Plan activities that you can do after meals to help you tolerate the distress if it arises. For example, play board games, play an instrument, watch a movie, sit with a family member, play with a pet, or engage with children or roommates.

2. Use a heating pad if your body is feeling uncomfortable. There are portable and disposable heating pads if you need to be mobile.

3. Be compassionate with yourself during this time. If your fullness resulted from eating more than you wanted to at a meal, or from a binge, allow some self-compassion for this journey. There will be ups and downs on a meandering path. It also might be helpful to assess with your therapist whether you experienced any binge triggers. Often a binge can be due to restriction, or an emotional cue like boredom, loneliness, depression, anxiety, or an event like an argument. Have a good "cope ahead" plan in a place.

Dealing with Stomach Pain Associated with Refeeding

You have most likely already realized that refeeding is emotionally challenging, and by now you've probably seen that it's also hard physically, making you feel worse before you actually feel better. And when motivation is low to begin with, it can be challenging to continue to push through.

You might begin to feel as if you can't tolerate gluten, dairy, or fats and may feel utterly confused as to what to eat. This increase in intolerance to food can happen because a restricted diet and malnutrition causes a reduction in the enzymes needed for digestion, including lactase (needed to break down lactose) and lipase (needed to break down dietary fat). The best way to increase these enzymes is to eat a variety of foods so they can be secreted and available. Digestion will improve as your nutrition improves, with time, consistency, and nourishment. *If you were not lactose or gluten intolerant before the onset of your ED, it is highly unlikely you are now.*

To ease some of the distress that you may experience during this time, you might find that adding a probiotic supplement is helpful. This is an over-the-counter supplement that can help restore gut bacteria. Lactase supplementation might also be helpful, but ideally we would want your body to produce its own lactase (though a supplement is helpful for anyone who is lactose intolerant). Antacids can help those experiencing burping, reflux, or burning in their chest. Such supplements should be used conservatively and discussed with your doctor. It may also help to minimize gas-producing foods such as the following.

- Beans (presoaking reduces the gas-producing potential of beans if you discard the soaking water and cook using fresh water)
- Vegetables such as artichokes, asparagus, broccoli, cabbage, Brussels sprouts, cauliflower, cucumbers, green peppers, onions, radishes, celery, carrots
- Fruits such as apples, peaches, raisins, bananas, apricots, prune juice, pears
- Whole grains and bran (adding them slowly to your diet can help reduce gas-forming potential)
- Carbonated drinks (these contain a great deal of CO_2, so let them stand open for several hours to allow the gas to escape)
- Diet foods, such as items containing sorbitol, and sugar-free candies and gums[10]
- Rice cakes, popcorn, rice crackers
- Bars that are high in fiber or in protein

It will be helpful during this time to reduce the consumption of fiber, fruits, and vegetables, which can exacerbate symptoms of gas and bloating. Your digestive tract is rebuilding itself and is fragile. Eating easy-to-digest foods and fewer fruits and vegetables will decrease symptoms and help minimize body image distress while allowing you to renourish without the extra discomfort.

"I have no idea when I am hungry and when I am full"

It can be exciting when your hunger levels return, but for some, these cues may not be noticeable. So, what does hunger feel like? You might have a sensation in your stomach, an emptiness, a pull, a throbbing. Your stomach might gurgle or growl, or there might be no sound at all. You might feel slowed down or tired. Or you might notice you are simply thinking about food more or becoming more sensitive to food smells. You might find that you are looking at food-related Instagrammers or websites or just talking more about food.

We do not expect your hunger and fullness cues to come back online until you have been eating regularly and consistently for several weeks. Missed meals, sickness, or gaps in progress can make it difficult to detect your hunger cues. Neurodivergent patients or patients who lack interoceptive awareness (the ability to assess, become aware of and respond to the body's signals/needs) might not experience their hunger and fullness cues even once they've recovered. It is common for many to rely on an external stimulus, like a schedule, to remind them to eat. It will be important to remain on a structured meal plan, with regular meals and snacks and to rely on external cues such as the clock ("It's noon—time for lunch") to know when to eat. Setting alarms can remind you to eat if you don't have a physical cue as a reminder. Eating regularly will help you stay on track. And this rhythm and regularity may stimulate your metabolism and typically increase your appetite over time.

Situations That Affect Appetite

There are many situations that can affect your appetite or ability to stay on track with your expected meals and snacks. For example, a breakup, the death of a loved one, a traumatic event, an injury or accident, birth of a child, divorce, the initiation to/withdrawal from/change in medications, sickness, change in living situation, the escalation of anxiety or depressive symptoms, and more. You may lose your appetite under these circumstances or find you are "stress eating." Navigating stressful circumstances can be disorienting, but staying on track with your nutrition is essential to help you maintain the strength, focus, and clarity to persevere.

Tips

1. **Recruit support.** It can help to confide in a few close people if you have them in your life so that they can support, motivate, and help you feel connected. It can be hard to be social when you're not feeling well or for fear of judgment from others about anything from your food to your body to how you look. It can also be hard to let others in. But mealtime accountability can make a huge difference in whether someone is actually eating a meal or engaging in ED behaviors. Perhaps you can consider eating meals, even a few times, with a close and trusted loved one? FaceTiming with a friend at mealtimes or planning lunch dates can help with added accountability.

2. **Have groceries delivered if it's an option in your area.** It can feel overwhelming during stressful times to go food shopping. Food deliveries are an increasingly available option. This can come with an added cost, so if this is not an option, consider asking a friend to help with grocery shopping. Yes, that means *asking for help!*

3. **Limit caffeine and alcohol.** Both can interfere with your ability to understand your hunger and satiety cues. This can lead to skipping meals, which can lead to bingeing or failure to meet your full meal plan (which can derail your medical goals).

4. **Self-care.** What feels good to you during this time? What do you need: a break, a bath, quiet time outside, a night off from cooking, a morning off from watching the kids, time off from work? Honor that. During stressful times, practicing self-care is never what we "want" to do, but it's often what's needed. See the self-soothing list at the end of this chapter (page 121).

The goal of course is to continue with your plan of 3 meals and 2 or 3 snacks. Is there a way to make this easier for you? Premade meals or frozen meals can be a huge help. Frozen vegetables, canned fruits, shakes, or bars, might be easier to grab. It's possible that during this time you might not be able to cook or prepare meals the way you had hoped, and that's okay. You might need to implement what we call "Plan B Nutrition." It means "whatever works." It might mean eating anything you can during this difficult time to avoid skipping the meal. And that's okay. Do the best you can. It's good to have a list of the foods that are your "staples" or "go-tos" that you can count on for a rainy day. Keep them on hand. It's hard to think straight when you are in an emotionally escalated state.

Quick Items to Have On Hand When Your Energy and Mood Are Low

Shakes

Carnation Instant Breakfast

Ensure Plus

BOOST Plus

Bars

Clif, Pro Meal, or Bobo's bars

Entrees

Frozen meals

Fruit

Cut-up fruit ready to grab in fridge

Apples, bananas, oranges—they last for a while

Dried fruit

Canned fruit, frozen fruit

Vegetables

Precut and ready-to-eat

Frozen veggies that you can easily heat

Dairy

Yogurt, cheese slices

Milk or chocolate milk boxes

Protein

Beef jerky, nuts and nut butters, pre-cut and ready-to-serve chicken, frozen meats (ready-to-serve)

Starches

Breads, tortillas, cereal

Mac and cheese, frozen rice/quinoa, corn, pasta, and couscous (all take a short time to prepare)

Frozen burritos, pizza

Fats

Butter

Nut butter

Salad dressing

Oil

Nuts

Shredded coconut

Chocolate

Avocado

Cream cheese

Sour cream

Snack foods

Ice cream

Chips

Pretzels

Lack of Motivation

It can be hard to persevere when it feels like recovery is filled with obstacles. You might think, "I just can't keep doing this!" So if you feel like you are losing hope, consider *why* you started your recovery journey and *what* motivates you. Take time with this; it will be a tool to return to anytime you're having trouble remembering *why* you decided to take the leap toward recovery.

Find Your "Why"

There are so many whys for recovery. What is yours? Here are some whys our patients have shared with us.

I want to get out of the hospital.

I want to be independent.

I want my period to return.

I want my testosterone levels to be higher.

I want my mood to be better.

I want to feel less depressed.

I want to be less anxious.

I want to feel stronger.

I want to stop getting injured.

I want to have children.

I want to meet a partner and put my best self out there.

I want to build muscle strength.

I want to have stronger bones.

I want to be a good role model for my children.

I want to be less anxious around food.

I want to be free.

I want to be more present for my partner, my family, and my friends.

I want to have better vocal clarity (I am a singer).

I want to have more energy.

> I want to travel.
>
> I want to move into my own apartment.
>
> I want to really start my life.

It could be helpful to explore the following prompts when exploring your motivation.

- How do I feel right now?
- How do I want to feel?
- How is the ED negatively impacting my life?
- What worries me the most about engaging the ED?
- What are my treatment goals?
- What are my reasons for recovery?
- What will I gain back in my life if I commit to treatment?
- Whom can I rely on for support when I need it?

Now that you've worked on your motivators, you'll need some tools to help you maintain your motivation when you feel it the least. Below is a short list of motivators we encourage you to add to and refer to throughout this process.

- Schedule a lunch date with a friend (either in person or over video).
- Keep your motivation list on the fridge and/or the dining table.
- Set weekly S.M.A.R.T. goals (S = specific, M = measurable, A = attainable, R = realistic, T = timely).[11]
- Create rewards for continued progress (a short vacation, a cozy blanket, a new book, fresh flowers, museum tickets; find what rewards you!)

Once you have a working motivation list started, it will be important to keep it handy. When you're not feeling well, when you're down about recovery, you can remind yourself of your goals and your "why" for recovery. Your treatment team will be a huge part of this process, there to help you continue to put one foot in front of the other. You will also need the help of your village. And when your team and your support system are not right there, you will want to practice pulling from your self-soothe list (see below) instead of engaging with the ED.

How do I stop engaging the ED? In chapter 12, Nan Shaw references a quote from Jenni Schaefer's *Life Without Ed*: "Disobey and disagree." When that ED tries to pull you in, you can disobey—do the opposite and rebel—or you can disagree and recognize "that's not going to serve me." Find what will serve *you* in that moment rather than what will serve the ED.

Below is a self-soothe list to get you thinking about what to do instead of engaging the ED. Look through it, add to it, and find what works for you. When the ED pops in, try one of these techniques instead. Then reward yourself for disobeying/disagreeing with the ED. This will provide positive reinforcement for listening to your healthy self and practicing self-care. And the more you practice self-care and the less you engage the ED, the easier it will be to listen to your healthy self. That light at the end of the tunnel will be closer with each step you take.

Self-Soothing

Take a warm bubble bath.

Take a walk outside (if cleared by your MD).

Find a nearby park or a spot in your yard to sit (or a window during colder weather) to feel the warmth of the sun on your face.

Call a friend or loved one.

Snuggle a beloved pet (or a stuffed animal if you don't have a pet).

Journal.

Listen to a favorite playlist or music.

Meditate.

Read a book.

Take a few deep breaths (inhale, exhale).

Stop to smell a flower, a scented candle, maybe even a pile of fresh laundry (again, find what makes you feel good).

What can you add to personalize this list?

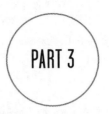

PART 3

Common Issues and Strategies for Recovery

CHAPTER 10

Getting Help from Experts and Loved Ones

PICKING UP THIS book is a great first step in seeking and receiving the support you need and deserve. While this book supports you in understanding your nutrition needs and shows you how to use the Plate-by-Plate Approach® in your recovery, it isn't a substitute for professional treatment but rather a companion to help you navigate treatment alongside the support of your village. Comprehensive treatment ideally involves a team of experts to guide you along in the process and ensure you are receiving the best care possible. It involves the support of those in your inner circle who will stay by your side throughout your recovery.

EDs, like many psychiatric disorders, are stigmatized. Studies show that stigma is more likely to lead to depression, negative self-esteem, distress, social alienation, social withdrawal, decreased physical health, increased ED symptoms, treatment avoidance, poor quality of life, and other complications.[1] Individuals with EDs have significantly increased mortality rates, the highest occurring in those with AN.[2] In short, those who are struggling with an ED need support!

If you're worried about what others will think when you share that you are struggling with an ED, it may help to begin by telling those in your inner circle first. Perhaps that's a partner, an immediate family member, a trusted relative, or a close friend. Those with EDs require huge amounts of support outside of their treatment team. It can be a grueling, exhausting, long, and bumpy road. This is your opportunity to find the person (or people) you trust the most and confide in them. Think about it: If you had just been diagnosed with cancer, who would you tell first? If you were going through a divorce, who would you lean on for support? If your child fell chronically ill, who would be there to help? It's likely that those same individuals want to be there to support you through recovery.

Who's in your inner circle? Begin to think about who you trust with information about your ED and treatment. Who can support you? Are there immediate family members, extended family members, friends, neighbors, people from work, friends from your place of worship or your sports team who can lend a helping hand?

Your inner circle can be helpful in ways you might not even realize! They can be there to help with meal accountability, grocery shopping, to accompany you to appointments, watch your pets, water your plants, answer your calls, text you back, FaceTime during a meal, keep you company, check on you, make you laugh, do nothing with you, hang out, or talk about something *besides food*. If your ED has caused you to feel isolated, and you've lost touch with your loved ones, it can be difficult to connect when you are not feeling your best. But connection is important to recovery.

"Where do I begin?"

In addition to your inner circle, you should assemble a strong multidisciplinary team of professionals to guide you through the treatment process.

1. A **therapist** to work closely with you, to guide you, and who can offer skills and support throughout the ED treatment process and beyond.

2. A **medical provider** to monitor your weight, vital signs, hormones, and lab work.

3. A **registered dietitian,** to guide you in implementing and utilizing the Plate-by-Plate Approach®.

4. A **psychiatrist,** if recommended, to assess whether medication may be helpful.

This team is your extra set of hands, and you'll build strong relationships with them. You should be able to trust them and know that they have your best interests in mind. The team will communicate often, sharing updates with your other providers to create a helpful plan of action. Your team should be on the same page with their messages to you so that there is no room for your ED to "split" the team or negotiate treatment recommendations. This will help you feel empowered and be consistent in your recovery. To maintain continuity of care, you'll want to meet with these providers weekly, biweekly, or at the frequency they recommend to best support your individual needs. This team of specialists will help you learn how to treat your ED effectively. They will continue to work with you for as long as it takes to make sure you have the greatest outcome in your recovery process.

When assembling a team of providers, you may want to find those who share your cultural background, exist in a larger body, or are part of the LGBTQIA+ community. You might want a provider who has had lived experience with an ED or other mental health concerns. It's important that you find providers you trust and who make you feel safe, heard, respected, and cared for. The process of ED recovery for adults is collaborative, wherein you choose providers to be partners with you in your journey. Here is a summary of each clinician's role in helping you recover.

Therapy

How do you identify an ED specialist therapist to add to your team? To begin, look at their experience. Ask questions specific to your needs. Look for certain certifications, including CEDS (Certified Eating Disorder Specialist) through IAEDP (International Association of Eating Disorders Professionals), or HAES® (Health at Every Size®), that indicate this specialty. The therapist could be at the master's level (LMFT, LCSW, LPCC) or a psychologist (PhD, or PsyD) or psychiatrist (MD). Many therapists in the field have gone through their own recovery, though this is not a requirement. The critical advantage of having an ED specialist on your team is to make sure you are working with someone who is familiar and comfortable with the interplay of psychology and biology. Such specialists are experts in "talking back" to an ED and are familiar with the many related issues of body image, body diversity, and recovery anxiety and appreciate that "what is healthy" is more complicated than any current fad.

A nonspecialist may not realize that health advice that is useful to someone with depression ("make sure you get regular exercise") could be harmful to someone with an ED who exercises compulsively. Equally harmful to someone suffering with an ED are culturally biased notions of weight goals, agreeing to a client's inappropriate weight loss goal, or accidentally reinforcing notions of food morality ("good" and "bad" foods). A specialist will be well versed in the ways an ED can "trick" clinicians into ignoring signs of illness, relapse, or obstacles to recovery. They know the paths to take or avoid and can advise you on specific ways to tolerate distress when things get hard. ED specialists have a good understanding of challenges to consider, such as medical events that might impact eating (oral surgery or a colonoscopy), life events that tend to overemphasize appearance (weddings and pregnancy), social events that require increased food flexibility (vacations, holidays, conferences), or other life events that can be specifically hard for those suffering with an ED. Of course, while each person's recovery is individual, it remains invaluable to have an experienced therapist to guide you.

The American Psychological Association recommends asking these questions when trying to find a therapist.[3]

- Are you licensed as a psychologist in this state?
- How many years have you been in practice?
- How much experience do you have working with people who are dealing with [the issue you'd like to resolve]?
- What do you consider to be your specialty or area of expertise?
- What kinds of treatments have you found effective in resolving [the issue you'd like to resolve]?
- What insurance do you accept?
- Will I need to pay you directly and then seek reimbursement from my insurance company, or do you bill the insurance company on my behalf?
- Are you part of my insurance network?
- Do you accept Medicare or Medicaid?

Medical

A medical provider will monitor your vital signs, hormones, lab work, and weight (if medically necessary). At this point, you may have already had a visit with your doctor regarding your health (weight, vital signs, etc.). Unless that provider is comfortable managing the complex medical needs of an adult with an ED, they will refer you to a specialist. The benefits of a specialized therapist also apply to medical and nutrition providers. Highly complex medical complications arise as a result of malnutrition, and these must be addressed quickly and be closely monitored to provide the best outcome. The messages given by a specialist will be very different from a nonspecialist. A low heart rate could be seen as "common" to a general doctor but is more severe in the context of malnutrition, insufficient nutrition, and an ED. A specialist can assess your lab work and determine the impact of your ED. These objective medical findings can be very helpful, but their absence doesn't mean you are not suffering. It takes expertise and compassion for a doctor to convey the details of an ED diagnosis.

A detailed account of what to expect from your medical provider can be found in chapter 11, which also covers "weight-inclusive health care," in which providers use markers besides weight as indicators of health.

A primary care provider typically carries one of the following credentials.

- Medical Doctor (MD)
- Doctor of Osteopathy (DO)
- Nurse Practitioner (NP)
- Physician Assistant (PA)

If you are already receiving care from one of these providers and they are unaware of your ED, consider making an appointment for a physical exam as soon as you can. Prior to the appointment, inform the provider of your ED so they can make the best use of the time. If you do not have a primary care provider, are you receiving care from other medical personnel? Perhaps an obstetrician-gynecologist (ob-gyn) who you see annually? Many medical providers can help direct you to the proper care once you inform them of your needs and goals.

Nutrition

Ideally, you will work with a registered dietician (RD) to seek guidance and coaching on how to use the Plate-by-Plate Approach®. The International Association of Eating Disorder Professionals offers a certification for dietitians that indicates extra training and credentialing in the field of EDs. This designation is "CEDS" (Certified Eating Disorder Specialist) or CEDRD (Certified Eating Disorder Registered Dietitian) and is a great added credential to look for when selecting a dietitian. Look for a weight-inclusive RD at ASDAH (Association for Size Diversity and Health).[4]

Just like medical providers, not all dietitians specialize in the treatment of EDs. The RD you work with will need a strong understanding of EDs and should work closely with the rest of your team. The initial nutrition visit will be mostly about gathering information—addressing and discussing struggles you have been dealing with in feeding and caring for yourself. A comprehensive baseline assessment will be conducted, similar to a set of questions we asked in chapter 3. While most of this initial session will include questions about your history, the RD will also be able to help you with the Plate-by-Plate Approach® and how to proceed at home. Toward the end of the appointment, they will also provide guidance about the initial stages of this treatment approach. You'll be expected to attend weekly or biweekly follow-up visits, with discussion about how meals have been going and what you're eating. The RD will then help create a plan for how to build on the previous week's progress. Throughout treatment, the dietitian will also help to reduce food fears and increase food exposure. This is discussed in more detail on page 168.

The dietitian may ask you to keep food records using a no-numbers app designed for ED recovery, such as Recovery Record, or Rise Up and Recover, or through their electronic medical record. Some software even offers photo tracking! These platforms allow the clinician to connect with you between sessions, as you upload photos and information (without discussing calories or other numbers) about meals and snacks consumed each day. For many, this helps with meal accountability, and the dietitian and treatment team are able to provide feedback on the photos. For others, keeping logs can be triggering, so food tracking might not be helpful.

Psychiatry

A psychiatrist may be recommended to prescribe and monitor use of psychiatric medications. You may also be referred to a psychiatrist who will perform an initial assessment and determine whether you may benefit from psychiatric medications if you aren't already taking any. While medications do not cure EDs, there are some that help manage ED symptoms and other psychological concerns (for example, anxiety, depression, or obsessive-compulsive disorder) should the psychiatrist make any additional diagnoses. You may have underlying anxiety or depression, for example, and medications can be helpful.

Every recommendation made by your treatment team is designed to help you recover as quickly as possible. Some recommendations may be hard to hear and difficult to implement. Your input on these decisions is important—sometimes what seems reasonable to providers might feel unreasonable to you. You may not understand why your RD is asking you to increase the amount of food on your plates or why your therapist is recommending that you bring your partner to one or more sessions. You may disagree with the psychiatrist's recommendation to start an antidepressant or the physician's recommendation to stop all physical activity. Good communication is critical during treatment, and it's important that everyone be on the same page. Feel free to speak up and express your concerns to the team.

You may wish to receive additional information from your team to better understand their recommendations and your options. Your treatment team should be able to provide you with sound, evidence-based explanations. You (or your ED) may become upset or uncomfortable during an appointment when you hear something you don't like, such as, "You've lost weight" (with the expectation that you should probably gain the weight back); "Your heart rate is dangerously low" (with the recommendation to refrain from exercise); "This is not enough food to meet your energy requirements" (with the implication that you might want to consider augmenting your meal plan); "We don't feel you are medically or psychologically stable enough to study abroad in London this summer"; or "You meet the criteria to be admitted to the hospital."

Remember, these recommendations, though difficult and disappointing, are made in the interest of helping you recover from an ED. Stay focused on what's best for you and your recovery. Allow your treatment team and those in your inner circle to support you during these difficult times.

Access to Care

EDs are associated with some of the highest levels of medical and social disability of any psychiatric disorder. Despite this, accessing treatment remains difficult for many, and insurance companies have historically offered inadequate coverage for necessary psychiatric treatment. If you do not have any medical or psychological providers, do you have an active health insurance plan (either private or government-based)? Are you covered under Medicare or Medicaid? If you do carry a health insurance plan, you can either go online to the plan's website and search "find a provider" or call the carrier's member access line directly to understand your provider options. If you're in an HMO, you will need to choose a primary care provider first and obtain referrals for ED specialists thereafter.

Based on your financial needs, you may choose to work with providers who are "in-network" or "out-of-network" with your insurance plan, or you may choose to pay privately for providers. ED treatment is expensive and can be cost-prohibitive for many. For resources to help you find providers, see page 303.

Taking Care of You

Feeding yourself 3 meals and at least 2 snacks a day, every day, when each meal is a struggle, can feel overwhelming and exhausting. After weeks or months of treatment, you may be asking yourself whether it is sustainable. Some individuals choose to take a leave of absence from their job during this time. Perhaps you took a leave and now that time is up. What do you do next? How do you get the help you need so that you can continue to fight for your recovery?

The first step is to talk with your support system and treatment team about how you are feeling. Ask those in your inner circle if they can pitch in to support you. Can anyone help you with grocery shopping and meal prep? If you live alone, is anyone able to move in with you for a while? Can you move in with anyone in your inner circle to allow them to help and support you? Are you exhausted from constant cooking? Perhaps you need some relief in meal preparation. If so, you may want to look into meal delivery services or grocery delivery programs that use an app to deliver food right to your door. This has the added benefit of adding variety to your diet. Quick and easy frozen meals might save time as well.

Self-care is also top priority when undergoing ED treatment. It can be helpful to create a list of ways in which you have historically practiced self-care, then build on that list for this time in your life. The following is a sample list, which you may find helpful as you brainstorm your own ideas.

- Take a bubble bath.
- Take five deep breaths.
- Listen to relaxing music.
- Meditate, on your own or with an app (Calm, Headspace).
- Play with your pets.
- Take a mindful walk around the neighborhood or somewhere calm and serene (e.g., the beach, a meadow, a park). Just be sure to check with your treatment team about exercise recommendations.
- Take a yoga class (if cleared medically).
- Read a fun book.
- Paint.
- Play an instrument.
- Listen to a calming podcast.
- Watch a funny movie.
- Drink a cup of herbal tea.
- Call a friend.
- Journal.
- Do a crossword puzzle.
- Play a round of solitaire.
- FaceTime a family member.
- Light a scented candle.
- Play sudoku.
- Laugh out loud.
- Fly a kite on the beach.
- Doodle.
- Take a scenic drive.
- Dance.
- Brush your hair.
- Shave.
- Change out of sweatpants.

Your village exists to support you, listen to you, and comfort you as you face what is likely to be the most challenging time in your life. Everything starts with recognizing what you need and being unafraid to ask for help. Don't be ashamed of your illness. The more you can share, the more support you'll receive. If you are struggling to find support, please refer to the resources on page 303 for more help.

CHAPTER 11

Common Medical Issues

By Lesley Williams, MD

EATING DISORDERS AREN'T always obvious. The symptoms can be subtle and easily hidden. Professionals, loved ones, and even the person who is suffering may not immediately recognize what is happening. Even when eating problems are recognized, there is a tendency to deny their seriousness. What may have started as an effort to "get healthy" or a way to cope with a difficult time can quickly spiral into a full-blown ED with serious medical complications.

EDs are not harmless. Your mental and physical health are at risk. We typically attribute the medical complications of EDs only to those who are at a severely low body weight. However, complications can occur regardless of a person's size. When you have an ED, it can be challenging to appreciate the toll it is slowly taking on your body and mind. This chapter highlights many of the potential medical problems associated with EDs, and it will help you seek care.

Medical Complications

Malnutrition

Malnutrition isn't about weight. Malnutrition is a broad term that refers to "all deviations from adequate and optimal nutritional status."

This can occur from specific nutrient deficiencies or inappropriate combinations or amounts of foods,[1] regardless of size or ED diagnosis. Not consuming enough calories for your daily functioning will cause the body to be in a negative energy balance. Once the body consumes storage calories to keep it running, it will begin to break down vital organs and tissues. Additionally, a body can be malnourished if it is taking in an adequate number of calories but the content of the calories does not meet the body's needs. For instance, someone who consumes solely candy may get in the total amount of calories required for the day. However, the type and variety is inadequate for their body's needs. As a result, they can also be malnourished and suffer some of the associated medical complications. Malnutrition simply means that the body is not getting all of the vital nutrients it needs to sustain itself. It is not a reflection of size.[2]

Malnutrition causes vital sign instability and is one of the main reasons for medical hospitalization. Typical instabilities include a low resting heart rate of less than 60 beats per minute (bpm), defined as bradycardia; low blood pressure with a systolic reading (the upper number of a blood pressure reading) of less than 90 (hypotension); EKG abnormalities; and orthostasis (inability to adjust heart rate and blood pressure appropriately with a change in position from lying to standing). The heart rate is assessed simply by taking your pulse in the office after resting. The heart rate is then measured in different positions, such as lying down and standing up, with the changes recorded.

Are My Vitals Unstable?

Check in with your medical provider to assess your vital signs. Ask for an assessment of heart rate, blood pressure, and orthostatic measures. You may or may not feel symptomatic when vitals are unstable. Some report light-headedness or feeling like they are going to pass out when blood pressure changes are too great. And some will feel overly tired/fatigued when heart rate is low.

Orthostatic hypotension refers to a drop in systolic blood pressure (the upper number) from lying to standing of greater than 20 bpm or a drop greater than 10 bpm in the diastolic blood pressure (the lower number of a blood pressure reading).

Orthostatic tachycardia refers to a heart rate change between lying down and standing up of greater than 20 bpm.

Bradycardia is defined as a heart rate of 60 bpm or less, and is commonly seen in patients with EDs.

Many people feel that their low heart rate reflects their athleticism, but this is not always the case. In the context of malnutrition, a low heart rate can be an indicator that your body is not getting enough fuel and is attempting to conserve energy by slowing things down—including your heart. When your heart rate is too low, you are at an increased risk of fainting, dizziness, irregular heart rhythms, heart failure, and cardiac arrest. The heart rate tends to go lower when you are asleep, and a low heart rate may require that you be hospitalized or wear a heart monitor so that your heart rate can be constantly monitored. The good news is that bradycardia will improve when you begin receiving adequate nutrition and fluids, and your heart rate will often return to normal.

"Refeeding syndrome" refers to a dangerous constellation of medical complications often resulting from aggressive nutritional rehabilitation. Low phosphorus, or hypophosphatemia, can be life-threatening in patients if not detected and corrected. Phosphorus is known to play an important role in cardiac and brain function. Phosphorus levels are in the normal range during malnutrition but upon refeeding can drop precipitously.[3] Phosphorus levels drop significantly in 27.5 percent of patients admitted to the hospital and typically reach their lowest level within the first week of refeeding.[4] A sudden drop in phosphorus can cause cardiac arrhythmias, and mental status changes that include confusion, anxiety, and irritability.

Cardiac irregularities

Heart issues can occur suddenly and have devastating effects for those suffering from ED. Cardiac symptoms include chest pain, palpitations, shortness of breath, and changes in vital signs. Malnutrition causes the heart to slow down to conserve energy, possibly leading to a dangerously low heart rate. Malnutrition can also cause decreased heart muscle mass. Low heart muscle mass makes it more challenging for the heart to pump effectively and can lead to heart failure and fluid overload.

The electrolyte imbalances caused by purging via vomiting or laxative abuse can deplete the vital electrolytes needed for the heart muscle to function. This can cause irregular heart rhythms, or cardiac arrhythmias, and even cause the heart to stop beating altogether (cardiac arrest). Regardless of the ED behaviors, proper heart function may be in jeopardy. Obtaining a thorough medical evaluation can help assess each person's individual risk factors. The first step in assessing the heart is listening to it during a physical exam and performing an electrocardiogram (ECG). Based on the findings, additional tests may be required to fully assess how the heart is functioning.

> ## Do You Need Urgent Medical Attention?[5]
>
> It is important to recognize that certain physical symptoms may indicate serious underlying medical complications and should not be ignored. If you experience any of these symptoms, you should seek immediate medical attention: confusion, seizures, fainting episodes, chest pain, blood in your vomit, severe abdominal pain or uncontrollable vomiting. Criteria for hospitalization can be found in the APA's *Practice Guideline for the Treatment of Patient's with Eating Disorders.*[6]

Gastrointestinal problems

Countless patients struggle with gastrointestinal (GI) issues that are ruling their lives. Sometimes it can be hard to determine if the GI issues lead to the ED behaviors or vice versa. Regardless of which issue started first, they are closely linked. It is quite common for those suffering EDs to experience multiple co-occurring GI symptoms. The symptoms can occur anywhere along the GI tract. The relationship between EDs and the GI system is further complicated by the gut-brain axis (GBA), a communication system of nerves, hormones, and microorganisms that takes place between the brain and the GI tract. When we feel something in our brain, it can impact how our GI system behaves. For instance, when we're nervous, pathways can be stimulated from our brain to our gut, which cause things to move through quickly, requiring us to urgently need to use the restroom. When people are malnourished or depressed, it can slow down GI transit and take food longer to travel, causing constipation.[7]

GI Symptoms Commonly Associated with ED[8]

GI SYMPTOM	EATING DISORDER CAUSE
Mouth sores	Acid from purging
Cracks at corners of mouth (angular cheilitis)	Malnutrition and purging
Gastroesophageal reflux disease (GERD)/Barrett's esophagus (pre–esophageal cancer)	Excess exposure of the lower esophagus to acid from the stomach, resulting in changes to the lining of the esophagus and ultimately leading to Barrett's esophagus and esophageal cancer
Gastroparesis/delayed gastric emptying	Decreased food intake
Constipation	Decreased food intake
Diarrhea	Laxative abuse
Hemorrhoids/rectal prolapse	Laxative abuse
Bloating/gas	Underproduction of digestive enzymes
Unintentional vomiting	Superior mesenteric artery (SMA) syndrome, or other GI issue, to be worked up by MD
Nausea	Decreased food intake
Abdominal pain	Inflammation of the liver from starvation or fatty infiltration, SMA, other GI issue

Endocrine irregularities

Hormones are the body's messengers. They send signals to our organs and tissues to help the body function properly. Our endocrine system is the complex network of organs that make hormones within our bodies. If hormones are not working optimally, it can cause serious health problems. Reproductive hormones have been linked to alterations in our eating patterns.[9] Additionally, malnutrition has been demonstrated to decrease production of vital hormones such as growth hormone, estrogen, testosterone, and thyroid hormones. Low hormone levels can profoundly affect your energy, libido, metabolism, mood, fertility, and eating patterns.

Obstetric/gynecologic problems

Emerging scientific evidence suggests that reproductive hormones, specifically estradiol, progesterone, and testosterone, can also play a role in the activation of ED symptoms.[10] The relationship between reproductive hormones and ED symptoms likely explains why puberty, menses, pregnancy, and menopause are stages in which an individual is more vulnerable to engaging with ED symptoms. There's still more to learn on this topic.

Menstrual irregularities

Irregular periods (oligomenorrhea) are common for those struggling with ED and are seen across all diagnoses. Periods might be shorter, missed, or lighter than usual and can be a sign that something is off. For those struggling with malnutrition since adolescence, the initiation of their first menses (menarche) may be delayed until adulthood (primary amenorrhea). Delayed menarche and/or irregular periods and associated hormone changes can lead to decreased bone mineral density (BMD) and osteoporosis. There are no set guidelines for monitoring BMD scans in patients with EDs. The typical practice is monitor any adult male or female with an active ED for six months or more, then every two years for ongoing surveillance.[11] This would be an indication to have a full medical evaluation, including having your BMD assessed. This can be done by having a simple imaging study done (BMD/DEXA scan).

Even if you are currently having regular periods, rapid weight fluctuations, calorie restriction, and ED behaviors may result in your period stopping for a span of time (secondary amenorrhea). Menstrual irregularities are typically a reflection of hormone imbalances. A medical workup is recommended to assess the presence of such conditions as polycystic ovarian syndrome (hormonal disorder causing irregular periods), hyperprolactinemia (elevated serum prolactin level), or anatomical abnormalities.[12] Besides osteoporosis, another common medical complication associated with menstrual irregularities caused by EDs is infertility.[13]

Birth control pills can artificially resume your menses. This does not mean that your bones are adequately protected. The menses resuming can provide a false sense of security that you're advancing in your recovery. The truth is that restoring your body weight and normalizing eating behaviors is the best way to improve your bone health. When your body naturally starts menstruating again, it is often a marker that guides the recovery process. Concern about bone health can be a great motivator for ED recovery. Your period resuming can be a great milestone to monitor and celebrate because it reflects that your body is healing and returning to normal functioning.

Lab abnormalities[14]

Several common lab abnormalities occur with EDs. It is also common for those struggling with ED behaviors to have severe illness and normal lab values. The severity of the illness is determined by the ED behaviors themselves, not the laboratory tests. Lab values are a helpful tool but don't always tell the whole story. If your labs are normal, it does not mean that you don't need help.

The following is a partial list of labs that are typically checked.

- CBC complete blood count
  - » Anemia
  - » Thrombocytopenia
  - » Leukopenia
- Comprehensive metabolic panel
  - » Electrolyte abnormalities
  - » Low blood glucose/hypoglycemia
  - » Low potassium/hypokalemia
  - » Low sodium/hyponatremia
  - » Low phosphorus/hypophosphatemia (part of refeeding syndrome)
  - » Evidence of dehydration (elevated blood urea nitrogen BUN and/or creatinine)
  - » Elevated liver enzymes
- Pancreatic enzymes
  - » Elevated amylase and/or lipase levels

- Lipid Panel
  - » Elevated cholesterol levels may reflect malnutrition
  - » Elevated triglyceride levels may reflect binge behaviors
- Thyroid Panel
  - » Thyroid stimulating hormone (TSH)—may be low, normal, or high
  - » T_3: May be low due to malnutrition. Assessment of T_3 and T_4 thyroid hormones is advised to fully assess thyroid function
- Hormone Studies
  - » Biological females: estradiol, FSH, LH, prolactin
  - » Testosterone levels
  - » Leptin (can be low in malnutrition)
- Urinalysis
  - » Specific gravity (measures hydration)
  - » pH testing for information on recent vomiting (high pH may indicate purging)
  - » Presence of ketones, which is a sign of starvation
  - » Leukocytes (infection) protein (kidney damage)

Infertility

Women with EDs have higher rates of infertility and poor reproductive health outcomes, regardless of the ED diagnosis.[15] When women struggle to get pregnant, they often blame themselves. They will put everything they do, especially their eating habits, under greater scrutiny. They see their diet as a potential cause for the struggle to conceive. As a result, they may start limiting their caloric intake in an effort to "get healthy and get pregnant." This can lead to weight loss and malnutrition.

As discussed previously, caloric restriction can cause malnutrition, which decreases hormones in the body that are vital to being able to conceive and maintain the pregnancy. Many women often seek treatment after they invested a lot of time and money trying to get pregnant. Each was dealing with different levels of disordered eating, from mild to severe. Despite their investment in multiple fertility treatments, the only thing standing between them and pregnancy was stabilizing their eating patterns. Once we were able to help them eat normally and achieve an adequate weight for their body, they went on to have happy, healthy pregnancies. This may not be the case for everyone, but those struggling with an ED and infertility should properly address their eating concerns prior to embarking on an extensive fertility workup

Pregnancy/postpartum

EDs are common during pregnancy and often go undetected.[16] The postpartum period can also be an especially vulnerable time for the development or reactivation of an ED. As previously discussed, people struggling with EDs often have menstrual irregularities. However, this does not protect them from getting pregnant. It is important to use contraceptive protection. Pregnancy can still happen, and an unplanned pregnancy while trying to navigate ED recovery is extremely challenging. Additionally, the body, life, and mood changes that come along with having a baby can be overwhelming for those who were previously in well-established ED recovery. Even if you are not struggling with ED behaviors during pregnancy, it's important to make your treatment team aware so that they can support you if struggles arise.

Midlife

Midlife is a season in which both men and women are more vulnerable to developing an ED.[17] This life stage is accompanied by multiple changes outside our control. ED behaviors can start as an effort to "get healthy" or deal with the unpredictability of this time period. It might sound like, "If I can control my body, then maybe I can stop these changes from happening." Having to navigate body changes, role shifts (at work and home), aging parents, family and friend deaths, health concerns, maturing children, and multiple other circumstances can cause an increased sense of being overwhelmed. During troubling times, we may feel that restricting our calories, overeating, or overexercising are ways to cope with what is going on.

Body image can also be significantly impacted during midlife due to potential changes in our appearance. As we mature, the ratio of fat to muscle in our bodies changes, even if our eating and exercise habits stay the same. As this occurs, the shape of our body may change even when our weight stays the same. We may also experience the "gifts" of hair loss/thinning, decreased skin elasticity, and so on. These are outward displays that "I'm maturing."

There are additional cognitive, physical, and emotional changes that occur with aging. Cognitively, there might be memory loss and a reduction in processing speed. Physically, there can be an increase in arthritis, osteoporosis, changes in libido, increases in erectile dysfunction, or vaginal dryness. There might be an increase in constipation, food intolerances, and reflux, making one's relationship with food change as well. Sleep patterns can worsen, as can mood, signaling depression, anxiety, and irritability. Interestingly, malnutrition associated with an ED causes many of these same effects, regardless of age. The combination of aging *and* an ED might escalate symptoms.

Dental/oral symptoms

Dental health is compromised by disordered eating in various ways. The acid production caused by purging via vomiting can erode the dental enamel. Bingeing, combined with poor dental hygiene, can also result in dental decay and cavities/caries. Additionally, the strength of our teeth, gums, and jawbone can deteriorate due to malnutrition. A thorough dental exam may also reveal ulcerations in the mouth or enlargement of the parotid and/or salivary glands from excessive vomiting, which can ultimately lead to tooth loss, a decreased ability to eat a wide variety of foods, and poor body image.[18] This can lead to the need for very expensive dental work and dental surgery. For more on medical, nutritional, and psychological factors to consider before thinking about oral surgery, see page 248.

Musculoskeletal symptoms

As we mature, broken bones can be life-threatening. Malnutrition from disordered eating can cause decreased muscle mass and osteoporosis, which predispose us to falls and fractures. The impact on bone density can persist even after you have achieved full recovery.[19] The best way to assess bone mineral density is to have a BMD/DEXA scan. This is an imaging study that can determine if you have had any bone loss. The DEXA scan is completed by the radiology department, but the amount of radiation is very low, just one tenth the amount of radiation in a standard chest X-ray. It is important for men and women who have suffered with an ED to have this scan. We can protect our bones by maintaining adequate body weight, engaging in weight-bearing exercise such as walking, and getting enough calcium and vitamin D.[20]

Dermatologic symptoms[21]

Skin is the largest organ in the body. There are a variety of ways it can be impacted by ED behaviors. Symptoms include dry skin (xerosis), brittle nails, hair loss, hypercarotenemia, and lanugo (fine hairs on on the skin that result from malnutrition; see table on page 20). Additional dermatologic symptoms related to an ED include the following.

- **Angular cheilitis:** painful inflammation and cracking of the corners of the mouth due to vitamin deficiency and/or irritation from purging
- **Russell's sign:** callus/scar located on the back of a hand and caused by teeth scraping against it during self-induced vomiting
- **Poor wound healing:** difficulty healing injuries
- **Acrocyanosis:** red/blue discoloration of hands and/or feet due to poor circulation
- **Pitting edema:** water retention caused by fluid shifts, laxative abuse, or low protein levels due to inadequate protein intake
- **Raynaud's phenomenon:** pale, painful, and/or numb fingertips with exposure to cold due to constriction of the small blood vessels/capillaries

Neurological symptoms

One common neurological symptom related to EDs is difficulty thinking and concentrating. Chronic malnutrition has been shown to cause brain atrophy and shrinkage. This can be seen on imaging studies of the brain. Electrolyte imbalances that occur from malnutrition and purging can result in seizures. Headaches and migraines can also be common. Vitamin deficiencies caused by improper nutrition can damage nerves and decrease nerve conduction. This can result in peripheral neuropathy (numbness or tingling in the hands and/or feet).

Psychiatric symptoms

EDs have one of the highest risks of mortality of any psychiatric disorder.[22] It is vital to recognize and treat co-occurring psychiatric illnesses when you are struggling with an ED. It is very challenging to work on nourishing yourself if you are also dealing with substance use, depression, anxiety, or other mental health condition. Even if you do not have a diagnosed psychiatric illness, you can experience psychiatric symptoms when you are struggling with disordered eating. ED symptoms can impact your mood and relationships by causing depression, anxiety, irritability, insomnia, mood lability, anger outbursts, and more. All individuals struggling with disordered eating should be screened and treated for co-occurring mental health issues.

Body Mass Index (BMI), weight stigma, and weight-inclusive care in ED recovery

How many times have you seen the BMI chart posted in your physician's office or had your own BMI listed in your medical chart? BMI is a simple equation developed by Belgian mathematician Lambert Adolphe Jacques Quetelet in 1832 as a quick way to measure height in relationship to weight (BMI = weight (pounds)/height (inches).[23] It was developed as a tool to determine the average weight for white European men. *It is not an extensively researched medical tool.* It was never developed to be a singular measure of everyone's overall health.[24] Despite the plethora of information to the contrary, physicians have historically been taught that BMI is a direct reflection of health. This idea can cause health care professionals to blame patients for their size and prescribe weight loss as the cure for all ailments. This type of stigmatization in health care settings leads to poor health outcomes for those living in larger bodies.

Weight-inclusive principles simply stated mean that people deserve access to respectful health care, regardless of their size.

ED treatment is typically focused on monitoring weight. An over-emphasis on weight has been demonstrated to be a catalyst for developing ED behaviors.[25] Many say the fear of being weighed or experiencing weight stigma deters them from seeking medical care. Weight should not be used as a marker of health. Incorporating principles from weight-inclusive care into ED treatment may be of benefit.

Weight stigma is defined as attributing negative characteristics to individuals living in larger bodies.[26] We live in a society that is very weight focused. It remains socially acceptable in most settings to demean those in larger bodies. Many people with EDs have personally experienced or witnessed weight stigma at some point in their lives. Quite frequently, the actual fear of weight stigma itself can be a contributing factor in developing an ED. Since weight stigma plays an integral role in EDs and affects the majority of those who struggle, it is important that patients and professionals understand and recognize it. EDs are not about weight. They are the result of eating patterns that negatively impact a person's physical body, mental health, and daily functioning.

Seeking medical care

Even if you do not have any obvious signs of the medical complications associated with EDs, there are many physical symptoms that may reflect a need for further evaluation. It is important not to ignore what your body is telling you. Even subtle signs and symptoms can indicate a serious condition.

Going to a physician's office can be an intimidating experience, especially for those who have previously experienced weight stigma in medical settings. Don't let that keep you from taking the first step. Knowing what to expect can help make navigating your medical visit easier. The first step is to try to identify a provider in your community who understands EDs and preferably has some experience with providing weight-inclusive care. Prior to your visit, do your research. You can start by walking through the office waiting room to see if there are any accessibility obstacles which may make your first visit uncomfortable. One of the first things that happens when you go to your medical appointment is that you will have your vital signs taken. This involves measuring your height, weight, blood pressure, temperature, and heart rate. You should feel empowered to ask for a proper-fitting blood pressure cuff. You can also decline having your weight taken if it makes you feel uncomfortable. Scales are often in public areas, and it is reasonable to not want your weight to be taken in front of others. Your mental health is important.

Being weighed at the doctor's office

Being weighed at the doctor's office can be a traumatic experience. Even those who don't struggle with eating issues find it challenging to be weighed in public. Many patients have even cited fear of being weighed as one of the things that keeps them from coming in for office visits. I have had people break down in tears or leave the office completely when it's time to step on the scale. If being weighed causes you anxiety, bring a "Don't Weigh Me Unless It's (Really) Medically Necessary" card to your visit.[27] It was created by Ginny Jones, a parent coach, and founder of More-Love.org, so patients can give their informed consent before getting their weight checked.[28] The card helps patients explain to their providers that "when you focus on my weight, I get stressed" and "weighing me every time I come in for an appointment and talking about my weight like it's a problem perpetuates weight stigma (a known and serious health risk)." Checking weight is necessary for providers when someone is medically unstable, has other medical conditions such as suppressed hormone levels, or when taking certain medications. We defer to the expertise of the medical provider, but it's important for you to know that your consent matters, and you don't need to be weighed for every ache and pain.

Case Study: Olivia

Olivia is a sixty-year-old Black female who was referred to me by the cardiology team for "eating issues." She has worsening heart valve function and the cardiologists felt strongly that if she would only "lose a few pounds," her health problems would go away. Olivia had been on countless diets over her lifetime. She was a perpetual "yo-yo dieter." Olivia was adamantly against the bariatric surgery her other doctors encouraged her to pursue, and she was sent to me as "a last-ditch effort" to help her make changes and avoid open-heart surgery.

What I discovered in my comprehensive medical assessment, which looked at Olivia's psychosocial history, was that she grew up in an impoverished family where food was scarce, and she used food to provide comfort in difficult times. I also learned that she was the matriarch of her family. Sundays were when everyone would gather at her home and she would cook delicious meals. Since the onset of the pandemic, those family mealtimes had ended and left a real void in her life. She often turned to food to fill that void. Olivia also revealed that exercise was an emotional trigger. Her younger sister had a massive heart attack while exercising and died just a few years earlier, and since that time Olivia has struggled to make herself engage in formal activity.

Through our conversation, it was clear that Olivia was struggling with binge-eating disorder—something other providers missed. EDs are frequently missed in Black patients and overlooked in those with larger bodies. Prescribing weight loss and bariatric surgery is not the answer. As a weight-inclusive, Health at Every Size medical provider, I worked with Olivia to earn her trust and to help her achieve her health goals.

Ultimately, Olivia improved. She found a therapist who understood trauma and disordered eating. She was able to slowly decrease her binge episodes and increase her activity. Her lack of activity was negatively affecting her heart more than her weight was. As she was able to move more, her heart function improved and she was less in the "danger zone" of needing a valve replacement.

Olivia's case reflects that healthy lifestyle habits are more important than size. She spent her entire life focused on decreasing her size. She thought that achieving that would mean that she had achieved health. Olivia lost and gained weight time and time again, and her health continued to decline. She was frustrated. Her doctors were frustrated. Her heart was failing. Everyone was focused on making her smaller. Her success hinged on her ability to put the quest for weight loss aside and just focus on her health. Evidence suggests that healthy habits are more important than weight loss in decreasing mortality.[29] In fact, large weight fluctuations have been linked to poorer cardiovascular outcomes over time.[30]

Weight-inclusive management of eating disorders

Despite the prevalence of EDs among people with a higher weight, they are frequently underrecognized and undertreated in this population.[31] Weight stigma is likely a contributing factor to this disparity. It is vital to incorporate size-inclusive principles into ED management to ensure that everyone suffering has access to equitable care. Historically, weight has been the primary outcome measured to track recovery progress. Weight-inclusive ED management encourages clinicians to be mindful that complications of EDs occur regardless of size, and we should focus on the behaviors themselves rather than solely on weight.

Recommendations for people with EDs who are at a higher weight seeking ED treatment[32]

1. Make sure your providers are comfortable collaborating with other professionals from different disciplines.

2. Always request psychotherapy as the first-line treatment for EDs.

3. Request non-dieting principles and interventions.

4. Recognize that addressing malnutrition and poor-quality diet is essential regardless of body size.

5. Be open to learning more about psychotropic medications with evidence in the treatment of EDs.

6. Ensure that physical activity focuses on positive physical and mental health benefits rather than changing body weight or shape.

7. Seek out exercise instructors with experience working with patients with larger bodies and EDs.

8. Include your family and support network in the process, so they can learn how conversation around bodies and eating can negatively affect you.

9. Avoid providers who use stigmatizing language, and don't be afraid to speak up.

Is My Doctor's Office Weight-Inclusive?[33]

-   Does the office treat the whole patient, offering symptom-specific solutions, without focusing on dieting and weight loss?
-   Ask the office: What kind of diversity, equity, and inclusion training does the staff have? Are they comfortable taking care of patients of various ages, sizes, sexual orientations, and cultures?
-   Is the physical environment welcoming to all people? Do the artwork, marketing materials, and staff members reflect a wide array of diversity?
-   Are the waiting room chairs big enough to accommodate all bodies?
-   Does the medical equipment accommodate all sizes (chairs, BP cuffs, gowns, exam tables, scales, etc.)?
-   How does the office handle it when a patient doesn't want to be weighed?
-   Where are patient weight checks conducted?

Eating disorders in marginalized groups

Simply stated, being marginalized means that you are not a part of the "in crowd." Feeling like you don't belong because of your difference can make you susceptible to developing an ED. If you belong to a marginalized group, the fact that you don't fit the typical ED image can also decrease the chances that your ED will be quickly recognized and addressed. We have emphasized many times in this chapter that EDs come in all shapes, colors, and sizes. Some concerns I repeatedly hear from patients with marginalized backgrounds are as follows.

1. The mental health impact of constantly feeling left out is not addressed.

2. No one ever asks how they cope with feeling different.

3. They are rarely screened for ED behaviors.

4. They are only asked about eating when their weight is considered above average.

5. The trauma of marginalization is not understood.

6. Their family didn't believe they had a problem.

Seeking help can be frightening and overwhelming. It may feel easier to ignore the problem than to act. Failing to address the ED can result in myriad medical complications, such as its worsening severity and extending the course of treatment. Reaching out to your primary care provider or ED specialist is typically the best first step in this process. Be advised that medical education on EDs is limited. Your PCP may not have all the answers, but it is important that they are willing to listen and learn.

CHAPTER 12

Exploring Therapeutic Strategies for Recovery

By Nan Shaw, LCSW, FBT, CEDS-S

The Role of Therapy in Recovery

In addition to pursuing physical recovery and nutritional rehabilitation, it is crucial to also address the thoughts, beliefs, emotions, and behaviors that maintain an ED and interfere with normal daily functioning in your life. Stabilizing weight, increasing food variety, or stopping purging do not equal freedom from an ED or absolute prevention of a relapse. Changing behaviors is where we need to start. EDs are about more than food and weight. EDs have a strong psychological component, with predictors of good treatment outcomes, including motivation, improved mood, reduced preoccupation with weight/shape, better interpersonal functioning, and greater self-compassion.[1] These are the purview of therapy.

EDs have been described as "emotion management disorders," recognizing that for ED sufferers, "starving numbs, bingeing soothes, and purging provides relief." In addition, they are "emotion converters" wherein "feelings like anger, fear, sadness, or shame get converted into thoughts of 'I feel fat' or 'I must run, purge, binge, and restrict more!'"[2] EDs can also be considered "(life) appetite thieves." They steal expected milestones from you, try to convince you that conflicts are unfixable and goals unachievable, and rob you of opportunities to build the life you want. How things started for you at the onset of the ED may morph into other notions about how the ED "helps" you. Addressing these psychological aspects are essential to ED treatment and recovery.

This is where working with an outpatient ED therapist comes in, whether meeting with you individually and/or with your family and loved ones. The general goals of therapy are to establish health and nutrition stability, build a life outside the ED, understand the ways the ED may have served you, and start to meet those needs differently or shift your needs completely. The goal is to achieve a life in which who you are and what you value is more important than a number on the scale, the food you eat, the miles you run, or the meals you avoid. The goal is a life that has you excited about things unrelated to your body's weight, shape, or appearance, and one in which you can successfully cope without starving, bingeing, purging, or compulsively exercising; a life that can make space for valuing appearance and self-care but refuses to overvalue them to the exclusion of all else. Breaking all the ED "rules" becomes key to defining your own set of guidelines to living life on your terms.

Recovery helps you navigate and evaluate your day in whole new ways, like focusing on how present you feel with your kids or how productive you feel at work or what kind of friend you strive to be. What to wear that day becomes a question of comfort and style and not self-worth. Meals become reasons to fuel, enjoy, socialize, and relax. Once no longer buffeted constantly by your ED, you can start to pursue your true "appetites" and manage your emotions. Therapy seeks to help you recalibrate and reconstitute the many ways your ED has taught you to assess yourself and schedule your time.

In her book *Life Without Ed*, Jenni Schaefer writes about "Disobey and Disagree," beautifully describing the importance of each in your recovery. Starting with disobeying the ED is legitimate and important to your recovery, during which time you *act* differently (for example, eating dinner even if your ED thinks you shouldn't). But actually disagreeing with the ED, during which you *act and think* differently, is where greater freedom arrives (you eat dinner because you know it's right for you and you want to). This is where you change your behaviors *and* your beliefs—and use therapy to help you get there.

How Do You Know You're Ready?

What "ready" looks like can be different for different people. Ultimately, *you* will know best when *you* are ready. Even by reading this book, you are likely contemplating nourishing yourself to a healthy place. Being "recovery curious" can be an important step toward being "recovery committed." You can be open to "disobey" (eat differently) while aiming to also "disagree" (think differently). Are you ready? How do you know if you're ready?

Readiness is not just a fearless resolve to throw out the ED no matter what, which can happen but isn't the only version of "ready" required). Readiness can also come from no longer enjoying what the ED offers you and feeling oppressed by its many rules. Readiness could show up as knowing you want "out," but feeling stuck about how to escape. It is feeling scared that life without your ED may be worse than being captive in it (it isn't). It is a recognition that how the ED is dictating how you spend your time and energy is hurting you and, perhaps, those around you. You can be ready if you want to change for others, because you love them or because they are scared for you or if you are trying to get pregnant and your ED is the main obstacle. You can be ready because your coach has told you not to play until you are healthy. Start where you can and build from there. This is what we mean by "building" a life you want for yourself. Just like the ED developed in pieces, you can dismantle it one brick at a time.

And, while ready, you may find yourself in apparent conflict with your team ("I want to go on that trip" or "I insist on continuing with my food avoidance, my exercise regimen, my body checking, etc.") These are the times to appreciate that your team is arguing with your ED on behalf of your recovery. They are arguing for you, not with you. Your team has been hired to save your life and set you free, and they take that role seriously. While your motivation to recover may ebb and flow, your team's commitment to you does not. Talk about this openly with your providers. EDs thrive on secrecy, and being honest with your team keeps that secrecy in check. If you have a history of treatment as a child or teen, you may approach therapy as an adult with some vestiges of the idea that therapy is something done "to you" versus "with you."

Therapy as an adult is a partnership with your providers. Again, make your past experience something you talk about with your therapist and team. Just like the medical and nutritional appointments are "biofeedback" on how things are going physically and nutritionally, therapy offers you feedback on your motivation, thoughts, feelings, and behaviors. It's not a judgment, it's merely information. Living with an ED can be like walking on a broken leg and wondering why it doesn't heal. Your team is responsible for reminding you that you need to keep the cast on, use the crutches, do the PT, give your body time and resources to heal, and be patient.

If you're not sure about your readiness, and for therapy specifically, don't fret. Try making an honest list of pros and cons of staying in your ED, and pros and cons of recovery and treatment. Really check in with yourself about your willingness and don't be put off by fear and worry. If this were easy, you would have done it already. Being scared doesn't mean, in this case, "don't do it." It just means it's hard to take this step, and it's hard to not know the exact outcome. But we do so many things without a guarantee. We do so because we have to, because we want more/better, and because healing is better than staying in suffering, even if we don't know the exact outcome. We keep the cast on, even if it's uncomfortable. I have never known a single person to regret their full recovery, but I sadly know too many people who regret their ongoing suffering.

What if you decide you are not ready to do anything, but you are interested in *thinking* about recovery? Approaching change happens in phases, during which we might initially acknowledge "something is off" before actually doing anything about it. One model nicely summarizes what those stages can look like.[3]

- Precontemplation (not even thinking there's a problem)
- Contemplation (thinking there may be a problem)
- Action (doing something about the problem)
- Maintenance (keeping up recovery)

Contemplating change is an important step and is very often time-consuming. It is the stage in which we, or those around us, are aware of our problematic eating, exercise, or body checking behaviors. We have thoughts like, "I don't want to think about food so much" or "I know how upsetting my restaurant avoidance is for my partner." We start to wonder about the cost of keeping the ED in our lives versus trying something else. This thinking sets us up for the "action" phase that comes next. Of course, the longer we contemplate recovery, the longer we suffer with the ED and its consequences. That said, good outcomes are still possible even without the gift of an earlier intervention (depending on diagnosis, severity of illness, and other factors). Point being: It is worth trying to recover whenever you're ready.

Therapists can support you in your contemplation, but typically only up to a point when "contemplating" seems to be less about exploring and establishing readiness and more about delaying and avoiding. This is not meant as a judgment. It merely acknowledges that action is required to recover. You cannot "audit" recovery. Therapists ultimately want to teach you to swim, not remain your lifeguard. Recovery is a *process*, not a *procedure*. It's not one-and-done. Your recovery requires time and your active engagement in changing how you eat, exercise, and cope, all the while fighting your ED's arguments against these very changes. It's not easy and takes time. But recovery doesn't require you to go it alone: Your team is there with you.

So, if you are contemplating recovery, as part of writing your list of pros and cons of illness and pros and cons of recovery (do it, don't just think about it) it might be helpful to explore the costs of illness and your specific fears around treatment. Why do you want to recover now? What might be the "whys" of recovery for you? What might be the obstacles? Many adults approach, or avoid, treatment because they feel it is all about gaining or losing weight, and while weight metrics are part of the equation of successful treatment, they are just a small part.

It's important to broaden the lens to take in all that you are hungry for in your life. I bet you'll discover that your dreams stretch beyond "managing my weight" or "just eating differently." Ask yourself, or discuss with your therapist: What is the cost of the ED in your life? What are you missing in your life that you want back? Is it your heart health, bone density, social life, fertility, joy, general health, being fully present, loving yourself, brain function, ease of activity, honesty, intimacy? Even identifying these answers can offer incredible insight and motivation to find your way out of the ED. Keep them handy. Remind yourself of them when recovery seems hard.

Sometimes patients feel stumped about where else their appetite leads them, as this focus has been eclipsed for so long. A client in this circumstance might confess, "I don't know what I want." Another way to find your "why" is by asking yourself, "What is the problem I'm trying to fix?" You might begin with, "I have a problem with food," then discover that it is actually a barrier to being as active as you'd like, or a problem with self-acceptance, food/nutrition, security, loneliness, mood, or internalized oppression. Culturally, we are quick to blame ourselves, our weight, or what we eat, and therapy seeks to expand the dialogue to the full context of your life and experience. For example, I had a client who complained of "having no motivation to exercise." In our work, it became clear she was nervous about going to her gym at night because the parking garage was blocks away and she felt unsafe walking alone. This was not a motivation problem. You may not immediately know the answers to what you are trying to fix, but stay curious, not critical. This will help you determine what actions to take.

Different Therapies, Shared Assumptions

You may have noticed a tendency to talk about the ED as if it is separate from you—to "externalize" the ED. This is part of many therapeutic approaches and informs the skill of "disobey and disagree." The language that "your eating disorder wants you to believe such and such" highlights the separation of you and your values from the ED. It allows for your "healthy self" to have a place at the table, and respectfully gives voice to parts of you that tend to get lost in chaos of the ED, such as the parts of you that are scared or agree with your treatment team, even when it doesn't seem that way. It also helps your loved ones to distinguish their upset and anguish at the ED, not at you, just as we might hate cancer, but not the cancer sufferer.

Patients are clear, when asked, that they care way more about being present with their toddler than what size pants they are wearing, or are vastly more interested in preserving their relationship with their partner than a number on the scale. It is meant to help you step back and really appreciate the struggle you are in with your ED, hopefully with greater perspective and compassion. It is not meant to discount parts of you that are important and central (enjoying discipline in your life, being organized, or wanting to be your best self). It is merely meant to highlight the ways the ED likely co-opted those parts of you to harm you, not lift you up.

Most therapeutic approaches share other core tenets. Different strategies might highlight different aspects of treatment, whether focusing on managing your emotions, challenging ED thoughts and values, practicing different behaviors, interrupting harmful behaviors, offering alternatives to coping, or addressing brain function and medications. That said, they all share some core assumptions of what makes for effective treatment.

The crucial role of at least some motivation and treatment engagement

- The importance of working with a specialized and multidisciplinary team
- The importance of including (and supporting) loved ones/caregivers
- The need for specific focus on eating, weight, and related thoughts and feelings
- The importance of education about biology, nutrition, and mental health

- The need for medical and nutritional stability first and foremost
- That body diversity is real and should be honored (in diagnosis and treatment)
- That "what is healthy" is specific to individuals and broader than just physical health
- That no one causes or chooses an ED (although we do choose treatment)
- That anyone can get an ED
- The importance of practicing self-compassion
- That we shouldn't believe everything we think (thoughts are not facts)
- That you are likely to feel worse before you feel better (emotionally and/or physically)
- A preference for being treated in the "least restrictive environment" possible
- That medications may have a role
- That change is absolutely possible!

Regardless of which therapeutic doors you walk through, you will hear these underlying tenets, find overlap, and choose the approaches that get you where you want to go.

Main Types of Therapies

As a way of introduction, I will describe some of the main outpatient therapies you may learn about as you pursue treatment for your ED. Some of these are well documented in their effectiveness, and others are in the early stages of application. While I use "eating disorders," it should be noted that some of these therapies may be more targeted to one diagnosis versus all EDs. These approaches are not mutually exclusive, often coexisting and overlapping. Furthermore, this list is not all-inclusive, nor is it meant to imply that you need to decide on one over another. These are approaches I've found to be clinically useful in helping patients break free from their ED and find their own "activist" stance. That stance proudly proclaims to their ED, once and for all, "I don't care about what you care about!" They involve tools of perspective, compassion, values, and practice, and the humor and grace to mess up. Each of these approaches involves more than the summary descriptions here. Think of this as an "appetizer" to the full buffet of treatment options that exist. Work with your team to help you identify where to start when it comes to therapy.

In general, most approaches discussed here share the starting goal of reducing immediately harmful symptoms (malnutrition, purging, binge eating, medical instability) and afterward focusing on thoughts, moods, behaviors, or interactions that maintain the ED, as well as managing painful, underlying emotions. Some approaches are delivered individually, some with family/support persons or in groups, and even some in combinations.

Family-based therapy

Before delving into the individual therapy options, let's talk briefly about family therapy. Family-based therapy (FBT) led the shift in viewing caregivers of those with EDs as valuable resources to tap. Originally developed for adolescents, FBT has shown promise in treating young adults, with some adjustments that acknowledge young adults' developmental stage and need for agency and autonomy.[4] These adjustments include "the amount of control parents take over the refeeding process, as well as the involvement of social support systems outside of just parents," along with issues of consent, confidentiality, acceptability of treatment, and a greater role for adjunctive individual sessions.[5]

Eva Musby has a great illustration of this shift from adolescent FBT, in which parents need to take the lead in getting their child out of the ED "hole," to young adult FBT, in which parents are invited to assist as the young adult begins to climb out of the hole on their own.

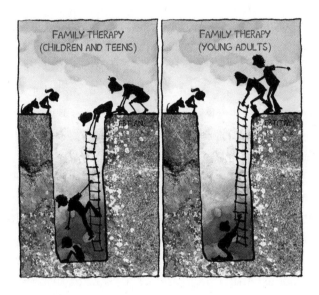

The purpose of actively including support persons in treatment is its tacit acknowledgment of the dangerous combination you face with an ED—that of lethal illness and treatment reluctance (or rejection). It is about adding resources to a depleted, bullied, and overwhelmed system . . . you! The genuine assumption is that "you are doing the very best that you can" yet you remain ill and at risk, in need of support from others. There is no illness for which we would tell you, or your loved ones, that just because you're over eighteen, it's time to get better on your own! Please don't let your ED make suffering alone some badge of honor. No one should suffer alone. For adults, including a support person involves an explicit invitation from you, along with your consent for your support person to talk openly with your team. For support to be effective, everyone needs to be working with all the right information. Secrets are the currency of the ED; honesty and openness are the antidote.

As an adult, you may choose the support person with whom you are willing to work to better handle meal planning and/or prepping and supervision around use of bathrooms or exercise. This can be a parent, other adult family member, or others you identify. Interestingly, it has been noted that even given this choice, most young adults do choose to have their parents in this role. In addition, living at home during this time is associated with better outcomes.[6] The main point is to allow you to be "off duty" from fighting all the ED thoughts and fears alone, instead choosing to invite your support person to help manage the myriad choices that swirl around food, exercise, and body checking. This is more like having a guardian angel than being "watched like a hawk."

As with adolescents, the ease of using the Plate-by-Plate Approach® is a huge benefit. Everyone in your support system can confidently use the same model of what/how much to eat without a lot of rigmarole or consultation. You get to step out of the arena with your ED and allow others to stand in and, frankly, stick up for you. Again, fighting *for* you and *against* your ED. Allow yourself this reprieve from the unremitting mental dialogue you have about what you "can and cannot" eat or do, and just catch your breath and rally your resources. It is not a failure on your part, nor is it giving up autonomy. It's simply inviting the cavalry to come to your aid until you feel strong enough to rejoin the battle.

Individual Therapies

After addressing immediate requirements of medical and nutritional stability, the focus of individual therapy can be on the thoughts, moods, emotion processing, behaviors, values, relationships and/or psychological and relational history that contribute to the onset and maintenance of your ED. Some therapy approaches may be more supportive and exploratory of the past/present/future. Others may be more geared to learning and practicing new skills, and some might be more symptom-targeted therapies. Some therapists will provide a combination of approaches. Following are some of the therapies you might learn about as you pursue options for yourself. Detailing each is beyond the scope of this chapter, but here are a few highlights to explain how they seek to provide a path out of the ED.

Cognitive behavioral therapy (CBT)

In general, CBT approaches offer skills to identify our negative self-talk and beliefs (that's the "cognitive" part), and then learn ways to question and/or counter them. It links our self-talk with how we feel and how we behave (that's the "behavioral" part) and provides various skills to shift these. CBT skills are ways of thinking and acting that shift our emotions and our ability to manage our emotions. CBT suggests we pay closer attention to how we talk to ourselves and be curious about our perceptions (where is the "evidence" of what I believe?). It can open our eyes to the nature of our self-dialogue and how distorted and mean our beliefs can be. Through CBT, we can begin to alter our self-talk, our behaviors, and how we feel as a result.

Cognitive behavioral therapy for EDs (CBT-ED) refers to therapies that use forms of general CBT, but with strategies and language designed specifically for those struggling with EDs, such as the role of changing nutrition behaviors to change thoughts and emotions underlying the ED.[7] One of the better known of these is enhanced cognitive behavioral therapy (CBT-E), which was developed by Christopher Fairburn, initially to treat bulimia nervosa and later to treat other EDs. The term "enhanced" again refers to those strategies geared for treating ED sufferers—specifically, overvaluation and control of shape/weight, as well as issues of perfectionism, low self-esteem, and interpersonal difficulties.[8]

An example might be the thought, "I hate my body," which I'm sure loved ones have tried to tell you is a totally unfair belief. CBT would have you consider a fairer and more open view, such as "I'm having a hard time with my body image right now," and even to consider adding, "but I'm not sure I can trust my opinion about my body." Can you imagine the difference in your mood and your subsequent actions if you could be fairer with your self-talk?

Another easy-to-use CBT skill to take the sting out of painful and biased thoughts is to add "maybe," "yet," or "prefer" to our language. "*Maybe* I'm being too critical," "I don't love my body *yet*," or "I would *prefer* to have more body compassion." Simple but powerful CBT tools you can use anywhere, anytime.

One of the things I say about some CBT skills is that they may feel insufficient compared to your suffering, but do not underestimate their power, as well as the power of even a small degree of change. For example, consider the behavior of breathing into a paper bag when hyperventilating. If you've ever experienced panic, breathing into a paper bag seems woefully inadequate to the intensity of your experience, but it works! This brings us to the other part of CBT, addressing behaviors, and how that can be equally influential in shifting ED habits. This could include paying attention, good sleep hygiene and mindful movement, and targeted exercises that "throw a wrench in the works" of your ED.

EDs are an illness of opportunity, particularly in early recovery. You are willing and committed to your recovery, but suddenly you "could" restrict, binge, purge, or move compulsively, and the temptation is high. Examples of "wrench-worthy" behaviors: If someone is trying very hard to not purge, they might consider taking their birth control pill right after a meal to add to their motivation to keep that meal down. Asking a loved one to go with you to a public restroom after a meal might make you less inclined to purge that meal. Avoiding known bathrooms in your environment that give you privacy to purge, declining the option of a private bathroom in a dorm, or taking off the bathroom lock so that your ED could get "caught." Putting your running shoes away might reinforce your goal of taking a break from running. Getting rid of your scale makes weight-checking less accessible. Any behaviors that support your recovery goals and make acting out with the ED even a little bit harder are worth trying. As a general rule, whenever you are too upset to talk back to your ED—you can't find the words or worry your words won't win against the ED—focus instead on any behaviors that will do that for you. Again, disobey (behaviorally) even if you can't in the moment disagree (argue).

Dialectical behavioral therapy (DBT)

Another skill-based CBT derivative is DBT (dialectical behavioral therapy) with its added emphasis on acceptance, mindfulness, learning to tolerate distress, and improving interpersonal effectiveness. Originally developed by Marsha Linehan for other diagnoses, it shows promise as an effective strategy with ED patients, in particular BED.[9] DBT seeks to offer patients new ways to approach difficulties by offering specific skills to increase coping with distress. It asks patients to compassionately question whether their ways of managing upset (for example, behaviors) work for them anymore by asking "is it effective?"[10] An example might be when a patient reports being upset about a coworker's comment and then using food to self-soothe, only to feel worse and deciding to purge. While patients initially feel "relieved," they also report feeling ashamed, depleted, and scared, with the original upsetting thing (coworker's comment) unchanged. DBT offers skills to compassionately suggest ways to shift this pattern to better regulate emotions, tolerate distress, and resolve conflict without relying on behaviors that ultimately hurt you.

The hallmark of DBT, particularly for black-and-white thinkers, is in the notion that two seemingly opposite things can be true at the same time. For example, you may know you are 100 percent committed to your recovery, while at the same time knowing you might relapse. This doesn't mean you are planning to relapse, nor does it mean your commitment is questionable. Instead, this means that we don't have to choose between "committed" and "not committed," instead recognizing the nuance of a commitment that at times may falter. Of course, we can falter in our commitment and still genuinely pursue recovery. By practicing this aspect of DBT alone, you can begin to experience fewer extremes in your thinking. One client told me, "CBT helped me argue with my ED, and DBT got me out of the argument altogether."

So, if problematic behaviors (like restricting, bingeing, purging, and excessively exercising) are attempts to help you cope with a situation or solve a problem but ultimately don't work, the goal of DBT is to find new, more adaptive ways to cope, particularly when you are in distress. Patients report greater urges to act on their ED during times of high distress and when CBT skills seem to be less effective. DBT's "distress tolerance skills'" are targeted skills for when someone feels too upset to use other skills geared to less intense emotions. When you're highly upset, being mindful can feel intolerable ("I am aware I'm freaking out!!") and "talking back to your thoughts" may feel impossible.

For this reason, I call distress tolerance skills "freak-out" skills, and they tend to be the opposite of the skills practiced to manage regular emotions—meaning, instead of paying attention to your thoughts or being mindful of your situation, you work to distract yourself from your thoughts and put your perceptions on hold until your emotions are less intense. These are considered "crisis intervention" skills. Once your distress is lower and your emotions moderated, you can again use CBT skills. Until then, "crisis intervention" skills are where it's at. These are meant to meet you where you are, and to acknowledge that when you are really upset ("I can't possibly go to that event, it will be awful"), you need different skills to bring us back to a baseline ("I'm a bit nervous about attending that event but I'll go.") Think of it like windshield wipers: When it's not raining, you don't use them even if you know they're there. You don't need them. But when it's lightly raining, you use them (CBT skills and emotion regulation skills), and when it's pouring, the wipers need to go super-fast (DBT distress tolerance skills). It's all about using just the right tool for the conditions you're in, without judgment.

Finally, DBT offers skills that directly address improving interpersonal relationships and supporting conflict resolution. This approach acknowledges how isolating an ED can be and how the ED interferes with your capacity to engage meaningfully. DBT highlights the importance of appropriate assertiveness and of being respectful of others as well as respecting yourself—maintaining "social health" alongside physical and psychological health.

Radically open DBT

A related and newer form of DBT, radically open DBT (RO-DBT), developed out of a recognition of the need for different skills to help those struggling with "over-control" (as many struggling with AN self-identify) versus those struggling with "under-control" (as many struggling with BN or BED self-identify). RO-DBT adds skills that focus on being *too regulated*, too rigid, and too risk-averse, as opposed to being too *dysregulated* as in regular DBT. RO-DBT focuses on skills to practice flexibility and openness, cultivating healthy self-doubt, along with more effective ways to socially connect. "RO-DBT contends that *emotional loneliness* represents the core problem for over-control, not *emotion dysregulation*."[11] Whereas DBT uses the notion of "radical acceptance" (letting go of fighting reality, dealing with "what is"), RO-DBT uses *"radical openness"* (challenging your perception of reality).[12]

Exposure therapy and exposure response prevention

Exposure therapy and exposure response prevention (ERP) are considered other CBT-informed approaches that offer patients experience and practice with behaviors their illness is having them avoid. The goal is to approach anxiety-provoking situations rather than avoiding them (e.g., *exposure* to a fear-food or to restaurants) and/or to interrupt the behaviors typically done in response (e.g., *response prevention*, seeking to prevent your usual response to restrict fear-foods or compensate for foods eaten). Exposure gives patients the opportunity to practice eating certain foods or portions, not purging after eating, or resting from compulsive exercise. With ongoing exposure and practice, the idea is that you can increasingly and successfully challenge your feared outcomes ("I'll get fat," "I can't do it," "I'll lose control") and prevent your usual ED responses (restrict, binge, purge, exercise). You learn that your ED's narrative of bad outcomes is wrong and overstated, meant to keep you scared and stuck. You learn, through experience, that what you feared and how you handled those fears were massively exaggerated in the ED. You realize that you *can* eat regularly, keep food down, have rest days, and that these are part of regular life and you don't need to be frightened. Exposure therapies are about doing, not talking about doing. Exposure therapies are also about doing routinely. Exposure requires ongoing practice until it's easy, even boring. It promotes not just "I can do it" but "I can do it with confidence, no problem." So, you may hear from your dietitian, "Keep having dessert until it's routine." And it will be!

Acceptance and commitment therapy (ACT)

ACT focuses on ACT-ing on one's values and can be used to highlight how those values are dissonant with ED values. It emphasizes the role of acceptance (like DBT) as well as commitment, and with the importance of taking action, not "auditing" recovery. It offers many exercises that help you explore what *you* want, and at the end of the day, to live your authentic life. What matters to you? What behaviors support what matters to you versus what matters to the ED? One ACT exercise has you imagining your eightieth birthday and who you'd want there. What would you want others to say about you? Would you want people to comment on your high value of weight and shape, or would you want them to talk about who you are as a person, what kind of friend, parent, colleague, or neighbor you are? These questions are explored with compassion, not judgment, in a way to make space for what YOU want.[13] Finally, ACT has you pay attention to your thoughts, as with CBT, but focuses on changing your relationship to your thoughts to be more compatible with your values. An example of this might be an awareness of thinking "I'm fat;" ACT would invite you to note, "I'm having the *thought* that I'm fat." "Thoughts are not facts" is a fundamental part of ACT therapy.

I have found that reconnecting with what is important to you and not to the ED is often very easy. Patients tend to have quick access to the awareness that they don't want their weight, shape, appearance to get in the way of their relationships, joy, or ease in life. There can be confusion and shame that despite this, they still have their ED. This is often the cause of the "stuck" feeling.

You may think: "I don't want to choose purging over hanging out with my friends, and yet I do. What does that say about me?" What it clearly tells you is that the ED is holding you hostage to things that are counter to your values. The discomfort gives you important information about this struggle and is not an indication of being "shallow" or a "hypocrite," as patients have worried. Use this discomfort to help set you free, move into it, and become curious about it. "This is NOT how I want to be in my life." So, the less-easy part, though doable, involves all the choices, behaviors, attitudes and actions that help you realign with your values. These have you practicing eating the dessert, choosing to be social versus alone in the gym, enjoying the dinner out with your partner, breaking all the ED "rules," disobeying, and disagreeing.

Group Therapy

You may also consider joining a group as part of your treatment. Groups can be psychoeducational, teaching skills like CBT, DBT, or ACT; therapy-focused; supportive in nature; and may involve meal practice. They can be open to all EDs, can be focused on one particular ED diagnosis, or highlight specific phases of treatment (early recovery versus relapse prevention).

Groups have some distinct advantages. They are cost-effective and offer a community of like-minded individuals in a venue that values open discussion without judgment. They challenge the isolation that can be part of having an ED, offering opportunities for therapist and peer feedback on particular ED and interpersonal struggles. Groups have been considered "social microcosms," mirroring how we are in our lives.[14] However, in a therapy group, we are given the opportunity to process our interactions and reactions in ways that real life doesn't usually allow.

Some groups are "closed," meaning they have a start and end date for everyone in the group. Others are "open" and offer frequent opportunities for new members to join. I have had patients find the support of being with others going through recovery essential to their own recovery. I have also had patients note difficulty in hearing of others' struggles or finding their own ED's desire to compete with other group members too distracting. Of course, this can change as your own motivation, and ability to have self-compassion, changes.

For loved ones, groups offer a particular path toward support and companionship on an otherwise lonely journey. As one caregiver told me, "Eating disorders are not casserole illnesses," meaning "people tend not to come by with offers of support or homemade casseroles." They simply don't understand it like they might with other illnesses. Loved ones report feeling heard, held, and helped in these support groups.

Other outpatient approaches might target your motivation, your somatic (bodily) experiences, movement, meditation, your family of origin and family systems, harm reduction, trauma work, role of substance use/abuse, brain function, medications, and more recently, use of psychedelics. This chapter is not meant to provide a thorough review of all treatments out there, but simply to offer an overview from which to start. Regardless of which modalities you and your therapist find the most useful, there are some common themes that come up for patients in recovery. In addition to questions of readiness, willingness, the "whys" of your recovery, and the inevitable ebb and flow of your commitment to change, many patients share other concerns about approaching therapy and staying the course.

Yoga Therapy

Yoga therapy is the application of yoga for health and healing. A yoga therapist is typically someone who is certified through the International Association for Yoga Training (IAYT). Yoga therapists complete yoga therapy–specific training and often also hold another health discipline (RN, RD, MD, etc.). A yoga therapist might focus on back pain, cancer, or mental health concerns such as reducing anxiety, stress, and depression or helping with body image concerns.

Sessions with a yoga therapist might combine body awareness, movement, breath work, and meditation or mindfulness with talk therapy. Therapists might use poses while talking through what it feels like in your body, mind, and heart (emotions). Therapists will work with you to address what you need. For example, maybe you need to bring your energy up that day, and so breath work would be helpful. Or maybe you are feeling depleted, and restorative poses would be helpful. For those who have high anxiety levels, calming the nervous system down with alternate nostril breathing could be helpful. But for others, relaxing can be difficult in an anxious state, and you might need to turn to active poses like "cat cow" to release excess energy.

"Yoga is about softening, not solving," says Suzannah Neufeld, C-IAYT, CEDS-S, author of *Awake at 3 a.m.: Yoga Therapy for Anxiety and Depression in Pregnancy and Early Motherhood*. When interviewed on the *Therapy Rocks!* podcast, Neufeld said, "It's an opportunity to greet what's there, without having to fix it. To have awareness and compassion. It's physically making space for what comes up, without any 'shoulds.'"[15] Yoga can provide an "intuitive listening to what's going on in your life." Can you work on something hard like a handstand without criticizing yourself? It can also be a practice in not giving up. Maybe yoga can allow for playfulness, joy, and excitement as you grow stronger and your skills improve? And, according to Neufeld, "sometimes we need to work on slowing down and allowing, not striving. We tune in to where we are out of balance. And sometimes, the feeling might just be that you're not feeling it today." Neufeld reminds her patients that the practice can be short, can be done anywhere, and requires little to get started.

She adds that for some the word "yoga" can be intimidating, and so she might ask patients to stretch or roll their hips around from side to side, or lie down and feel their breath in their body. It might be something that helps them to take time with their body to breathe and explore what they need.

CHAPTER 13

To Exercise or Not: Managing Exercise and Dysfunctional Movement

PHYSICAL ACTIVITY HELPS to improve mood, sleep, energy, longevity, and body image, and also reduces stress, anxiety, and depression. Yet, despite the many ways exercise aims to improve health, in the context of an ED, energy imbalance, or compulsive movement, the benefits of exercise can backfire. In fact, there is a higher incidence of EDs among athletes.[1] While athletes are known to be competitive, driven, perfectionistic, hard-working, and rule-following, there is often a pressure to succeed that can be self-imposed or encouraged by the team, coaches, or media. There can also be pressure for an athlete to conform to certain body standards. Athletes frequently compare their body to those of others in similar sports positions.

In this chapter, we will explore how frequent physical activity, paired with a limited or restricted diet, can have a negative effect on every system of the body and on sports performance. We explore a balanced versus an unbalanced relationship with exercise, and when to shut down your exercise program. While exercise is usually perceived as "beneficial" and "healthy," it can also be dangerous if you are not in a stable place in ED recovery. The decision about whether it is safe for you to exercise should be considered carefully by the entire treatment team, who can assess medical, psychological, and nutritional readiness.

RED-S: Relative Energy Deficiency in Sport

"Something feels off" is what we might hear from someone who exercises a lot when they come to our office looking for help. Those who exercise can be very intuitive about their bodies when they want to be. When they come to see us, though, usually there is something that has caught their attention. Maybe it was a few missed periods. Or the feeling of *always being tired*. Or *always being sick*. Or *always getting injured*. Three injuries later, maybe a light bulb goes on. "This isn't normal!" "Aren't I healthy?" "What's going on with my body?"

Relative energy deficiency in sport (RED-S) is common among athletes and in those who exercise and highlights the effects that even a small energy imbalance can have.[2] An energy imbalance means you are not eating enough to make up for your expenditure of energy and to cover your nutritional needs. RED-S can affect people of all body sizes, physical abilities, ethnicities, ages, and activity levels. If an energy imbalance exists, whether it's intentional (dieting) or unintentional (overtraining or an energy imbalance), every area of the body will be affected.

This energy imbalance has the power to affect all systems of your body. Athletes who are not properly fueling or simply can't keep up with their energy demands may find that though they train hard, they fail to improve—or worse, their performance declines. Sometimes their coach or family member may notice the problem first. In this state, the athlete might be slower, weaker, have less endurance, be more prone to injury, have a reduced training response (failure to progress despite training hard), be more irritable, and feel more depressed.

Even in a state of energy deprivation, athletes may initially see a temporary *increase* in their performance. This might cause them to think, "How bad could my eating be?" and reinforces the maladaptive eating and exercise behaviors that perpetuate the RED-S/disordered eating cycle. It's only a matter of time before the body begins to break down, showing signs of wear and tear, inflammation, and injury.

RED-S updates the Female Athlete Triad, which previously described a triad of reduced energy availability, reduced bone health, and suppressed menstrual function in females. Similar to RED-S, the Female Athlete Triad highlights the negative effects of eating too little for one's energy output, yet RED-S applies not only to women, but to men and postmenopausal women (older women who are no longer menstruating). RED-S also highlights the deleterious effects on many body systems, not just on menstruation and bone health. An insufficient amount of food, overtraining, or the combination of the two can lead to a state of "energy deficiency" (also known as "low energy availability").

For biological females, menstrual irregularities can often be a sign that something is physiologically off. While amenorrhea is common among athletes, it's not considered "normal." Alterations to one's menstrual cycle—particularly if previously regular—could be a sign of RED-S. One's cycle might be shorter, lighter, longer, or there might be missed cycles altogether. An energy imbalance can occur intentionally (due to dieting or clean eating) or unintentionally (due to a high training load, stress, trauma, depression, or anxiety). Biological males, who lack the marker of menstruation, have to rely on other markers of reduced testosterone levels, such as a reduction in morning erections or decreased sex drive. Testosterone levels can be checked through lab work.

An energy imbalance can occur for a variety of reasons. Notably, this can occur when someone restricts their caloric intake in an attempt to achieve a desired weight or body composition (more on weight goals on pages 179–80). Any situation that makes it challenging to meet your energy needs or to logistically ensure you are able to meet your full meal plan make a person particularly susceptible to RED-S. Examples include long exercise sessions, busy daily schedules, life transitions, changes in mood, suppressed hunger cues, stomach upset, or bloating.

A state of energy deficiency can also result from a large amount of movement throughout the day, not associated with training or sports. Often, athletes don't realize how active their life is! Walking to the grocery store, biking to and from work, hiking with friends on the weekends, walking the dog a few times a day, and playing pickup basketball are activities that can have an effect. You might be a talented, competitive athlete, and think, "Really? Walking the dog is the reason for my troubles?" And it turns out, in part, it could be.

Many think that if they are not sweating, the movement doesn't count. But that's not true. Long, frequent dog walks can easily increase energy expenditure—and if you are doing that several times a day, it begins to have a big impact. The energy expenditure associated with a dog walk (if more than ten to fifteen minutes) needs to be accounted for in your food intake or else an energy deficit will ensue. Similarly, standing can have a bigger impact than most realize. We had a patient who began working long hours at a café. She was on her feet all day. She changed nothing else about her food and exercise intake the first week and was surprised when her vital signs showed a marked reduction.

Food insecurity can also be a factor for an energy deficiency occurring in athletes. Some athletes skip meals to prioritize feeding their dependents or do not have access to the foods they need to sufficiently nourish their bodies.[3] Some athletes might be living abroad, where the food is culturally different; this has been seen in Kenyan runners,[4] with whom there have been "reasonably prevalent" instances of RED-S.[5]

Closing the Energy Gap

Correcting this energy deficit, simply by training less, eating more, or both reverses most of the associated complications and improves performance. Closing the energy gap allows you to get faster and stronger, to be less sore, to feel happier and healthier! Of course, this also applies to concentration and coordination. Many are so happy when their brain fog lifts and they have their full mental capacity back. It can be, quite literally, a game changer.

Increasing snacks or meal size or adding a supplemental shake, adding more rest days, increasing total caloric intake, and improving dietary practices in general can be helpful in closing the energy gap.[6] For some, once the energy imbalance is identified, they are motivated to close the gap between energy expenditure and energy intake. They come to realize that eating more will help them fix many of the medical and psychological side effects they have been experiencing. Others may carry a fear that adding more food will negatively affect their weight, their performance, or how they feel while competing. But as a person increases their caloric intake, their metabolic rate speeds up. This results in an improved metabolism, which is connected to improved energy, endurance, stamina, appetite, performance, training response, and recovery from exercise.

Some people can intuitively and naturally add more food. If your hunger cues are not obvious, you might not recognize that you need to eat more. Becoming aware that something like an injury, or change in season, can predispose you to RED-S is a great way to stay vigilant about your nutrition and take action to prevent it from happening. This can also help with the return of one's menstrual cycle and boosting testosterone levels. Regardless of why the energy imbalance occurs, the treatment is the same: Eat more, rest more, manage stress levels, and gain weight if needed. Here are a couple of considerations to prevent and/or recover from RED-S.

Nutrition

- Include all food groups (carbs, proteins, veggies/fruits, fats, and dairy or dairy alternative). Fill your plate and eat everything on it! This keeps meals balanced and ensures that the volume is "enough."

- Eat every few hours to stimulate the metabolism and keep the body fueled. Eating more regularly throughout the day has been shown to be beneficial in reducing cortisol levels, which can be helpful for the resumption of menses.[7]

- Add foods that contain fats. This can help boost testosterone and estradiol levels. Fats help absorb vitamin D, which is needed to absorb calcium—and calcium builds strong bones.

- Add extra fuel for added workouts!

Rest

- Take rest days at least once or twice a week. Examples of rest day activities include stretching, yoga, and short walks. You might "catch up" with food on these days, if you didn't eat enough on training days. This helps to suppress cortisol levels, which influences the hypothalamic axis, responsible for hormone production.

- Reduce exercising intensity. A study by Mastorakas et al. found that when training at 40 percent maximum intensity, there was no subsequent rise in cortisol levels. At 60 percent maximum intensity, there was a 40 percent increase in cortisol levels, and at 80 percent maximum intensity, there was an 85 percent increase in cortisol levels.[8]

Weight gain

For those who have lost weight, gaining it back is usually necessary. Weight gain is often a necessary step to heal the body, close the energy gap, stimulate metabolism, and boost estrogen and testosterone levels. This needs to happen even if you think you are at a "healthy" weight. A healthy weight *for your body* is unique to you and should not be based on a chart you read online.

Stress management

- Let go of the preoccupation with food and exercise, which may include tracking and measuring. Letting go of these behaviors can initially be stressful but can reduce the obsessiveness around food, numbers, and tracking.

- To help yourself unwind, meditate, play or listen to music, be in nature, or take a bath.

- Check in with a sport psychologist or your current therapist to assess your mindset and stress levels, especially throughout the grind of the season.

Hormonal tracking

- Track your menstrual cycles. Download an app (such as Period Tracker, Period Diary, or Clue) that will help you notice when there is a change in your cycle (length, flow, time between cycles).

- Note that periods can be irregular during perimenopause and absent once menopause begins.

- Check in with a doctor who can assess vitals and lab work to see if there are concerning changes.

- You might wish to talk to a sports dietitian to help you assess your energy balance. Look for a Certified Specialist in Sports Dietetics (CSSD) or a Certified Eating Disorder Specialist (CEDS).

Forty Factors That Affect Sports Performance

There is a belief in sports that weighing less will help you to perform better. Pressure to weigh in at a certain number or maintain a certain body composition can fuel dangerous and unhealthy behaviors among athletes. According to research summarized by Ron Thompson, PhD, athletic performance is affected by forty factors, yet many people are focused solely on weight. These factors include sleep, mental toughness, concentration, confidence, reaction time, rest, coordination, commitment, coachability, skills training, endurance, flexibility, whether the athlete missed a meal, hydration, whether they are following recovery protocols, and more. Yet there continues to be a harmful, unnecessary, overemphasis on weight, which is just one of many factors affecting sports performance. Forcing your body to reach a weight that is unnatural can be harmful to your health, suppress metabolism, and cause unstable vital signs. Performance can worsen by making you slower and less strong (muscle-building potential is reduced) while delaying recovery.

Riley Nickols, PhD, a sport psychologist and Certified Eating Disorder Specialist and Supervisor (CEDS-S) at Mind Body Endurance, notes, "Our bodies perform optimally and are more apt to sustain a consistent level of performance when physically, physiologically, and psychologically healthy. Specific to weight, our bodies and brain optimally function at a weight that is individualized, and most appropriate for our unique genetic makeup rather than attempting to modify weight to fit a perceived ideal."

Checking in with an expert about your goals can help ensure you are considering what makes sense for your body. Coaches and/or patients may assign a "performance" weight or a goal weight. It might be helpful to question: Where did that number come from? What is the cost for you to get there? Where does *your* body actually thrive? Usually, that is a place where exercise, food intake, thoughts about food and exercise, and food behaviors are in a state of energy balance and peace.

Unbalanced Movement

As with eating a "healthy" diet, being fit and exercising regularly attracts praise and admiration. Exercising in a mindful, balanced, and healthy way can slide into being all-consuming, obsessive, and harmful. Many people think that moving more is better, so it is not surprising that those who have dysfunctional relationships with exercise easily stay under the radar.

Approximately 50 percent of those struggling with an ED also struggle with compulsive exercise.[9] Excessive exercise has been associated with more chronic EDs, severe symptoms, and as a predictor of relapse.[10] Interestingly, there is no specified amount of exercise (duration, intensity, or frequency) that automatically flags someone's movement as "excessive." Factors such as one's training level, physical condition, age, and health status are taken into account when assessing whether one's movement is excessive *for them*.[11] There are also several qualitative characteristics pertaining to one's relationship with movement that might characterize their exercise as dysfunctional. For example, the relationship might become more compulsive, urgent, and distressing. An individual might use exercise to cope with painful emotions or to manage their mood. There tend to be rigid rules around how a person must exercise, and if those rules are not followed, the person will experience extreme distress. Some individuals tell themselves they can only eat if they can exercise, or they punish themselves for eating "something bad" with compensatory exercises.

Those who have developed a concerning relationship with exercise may train while injured or sick, or lose interest in their once-beloved sport and opt for something more intense. They may put themselves in danger by exercising in extreme conditions (heat waves, freezing temperatures), very early in the morning or late at night. When there is an unbalanced relationship with exercise, there tends to be a focus on weight, shape, or body, with an emphasis on burning calories. An interesting question to explore might be, "If exercise didn't burn any calories, would you still do it?"

A compulsive exerciser might do ten squats every time they pick something up off the ground or read while in a plank pose. They might be unable to sit still, might stand while watching TV, pace around the house, climb the stairs multiple times, or sit in a certain way at the table, so as to contract their abdominal muscles or engage their leg muscles. Additionally, there may be a high level of anxiety associated with missed practices or training sessions that can result in compensatory behaviors (e.g., restricting calories) in an effort to alleviate emotional distress.

Often, characteristics of being a successful athlete can overlap with some of the characteristics described in compulsive exercise, according to Riley Nickols. "Athletes are praised for getting in more workouts. Coaches love those athletes. These compulsive traits get reinforced inadvertently. What is unbalanced, and what is more normative for sport?" Compulsive exercise involves an obsession with exercise. We also see athletes training through injury, which has been normalized and which also occurs when someone is compulsive about movement.[12]

Two traits have been described to differentiate between excellence in sport and dysfunctional movement. One is flexibility. Can the athlete demonstrate flexibility by reducing training on weeks/days off? Can they taper their training between seasons and limit training when the coach gives them time off? The second factor is whether an athlete adds "additional exercise" on top of their training, with the goal of manipulating weight and body.[13] Or is the athlete able to prioritize resting their body? Dr. Nickols adds, "I never knew a coach that under-conditioned an athlete." Added sessions is a sign that something might be off.

	MINDFUL/HEALTHY EXERCISE	COMPULSIVE EXERCISE
GOAL	To challenge oneself and engage in a variety of activities that are enjoyable and energizing	To alter one's appearance and/or negative discomfort
PERFORMANCE OUTCOMES	Incremental gains	Plateaus/decreases
MINDSET	Work hard/rest hard	Move to move/rest is unnecessary
PACE	Athletes have many speeds, including very slow, and they use all of them	One gear only: fast/intense
ROLE	Exercise is only one part of identity and it is enjoyable	Exercise is the ONLY form of identity and activity is mandatory
APPROACH	Flexible and adaptable	Rigid
APPROACH	Curious/open to new information	Close-minded
APPROACH	Resourceful, driven, and rational	Compulsive and anxious
INJURY	Modify due to illness and injury	Train through illness and injury

Copyright Kate Bennett

Once the issue is identified, it's helpful to explore what is behind the need for someone to exercise in this way. For some, it might be anxiety or a desire to disengage from challenging emotions. For others, it can be to justify eating and guilt, or to serve as a coping mechanism.

Mindfulness is often used to enhance awareness around movement. Here, the person can learn to listen to their body to assess, recognize, and respond to cues of fatigue and soreness. This can be of value for preventing injury and minimizing overtraining.[14] Assessing how one feels is fundamental to understanding how to adjust intensity and training programs.

Exposure and response prevention (ERP), used in the treatment of obsessive-compulsive disorder, can also be used to reduce compulsive movement.[15] Using ERP, an athlete might be exposed to an exercise cue (watching cyclists or runners or swimmers training) and work to resist the urge that comes up for them to move. Athletes can use distraction techniques (meditating, calling a friend) to manage these urges. Lastly, studies have shown that varying exercise routines is associated with a greater intrinsic motivation and a reduction in exercise boredom.[16] Variety in training might be a gateway for minimizing the rigidity and monotony found in one's exercise routine, and for increasing joy.

Is It Time to Ditch Your Tracking Device?

For some, fitness wearables can be a way of improving performance. But tracking could be problematic for high-risk populations, including those with obsessive-compulsive tendencies, EDs, or those who struggle with compulsive exercise and their relationship with movement.

For some, tracking can lead to invasive and persistent thoughts about exercising more or thoughts of guilt about not exercising enough. Seeing numbers might cause a person to skip rest days or set unrealistic goals that increase the likelihood of injury. Tracking watches like Garmin send messages like "Detraining status," a nod that you are now in the "untrained zone." Or they message you to "MOVE!" or "STAND!" Some clients use multiple tracking devices to compare data. Some clients have felt tethered to the data—unable to exercise without the numbers.

For others, however, the data can help self-monitor and contain exercise. "The watch kept me honest. I was able to stick to my allotted intensity, as tracked through my heart rate, and duration, prescribed by my team," a client shared. Also, the use of heart rate variability (HRV) measurements can help assess strain and need for recovery.[17] A low HRV might mean it's time to take a rest day or encourage yourself to initiate more recovery activities like yoga and mindfulness.[18] What is most helpful to you as you try to find more balance? Here are some questions to consider.

- Do you feel guilty/ashamed for not reaching goals?
- Do you keep setting higher/unrealistic goals or go to extremes to reach your goals?

- Does the watch cause you to obsess or ruminate about movement?
- Can you shrug off the watch's demands to MOVE and STAND if you are not in the mood?
- Are you wearing multiple trackers because you find it hard to "trust" one?
- Do you struggle to take a rest day?
- Do you have OCD and/or an unbalanced relationship with exercise?
- Is your mood (and therefore workout) ruined if you are not able to have your watch with you?
- Does the watch make your mindset, medical condition, mood, stress level, or mental clarity worse?
- Is the watch helping or harming your recovery?

What does a balanced relationship with exercise look like? Exercise should be enjoyable and energizing, not exhausting or painful. Exercise is just one part of your life rather than the main focus. Dr. Nickols asks, "Do you structure your life around exercise or training for your sport, or do you structure exercise and training for your sport around your life?" In a healthy relationship with exercise, an individual should be able to vary the intensity of workouts, meaning that training can occur at a lower intensity some of the time and more intensely at others. Someone who is compulsively exercising may only know and exhibit one gear—high intensity, or near maximum effort—during workouts, whereas those who exercise mindfully can be more flexible. For example, if it's cold and raining outside, a balanced exerciser may decide to skip a run and opt for a cup of tea and a good book by the fire. Conversely, a compulsive exerciser will go out in the cold and rain, perhaps in the early morning hours when it's still dark. When nourishing one's body sufficiently, an individual who exercises moderately will often see incremental performance gains, whereas an individual who exercises compulsively will likely experience a decline in performance over time.

Case Study: Jayden

Jayden is a triathlete. She was doing thirty-mile bike rides and hour-long swims several days a week, plus running multiple times a week. She had a few nagging injuries. Though she had done triathlons in the past, there was no race on the calendar. Typically, athletes' training schedules are "periodized" around their race schedules, meaning their training increases and decreases to account for where they are in the season, allowing the body to rest and recover, reduce inflammation and rebuild. Keeping the exercise as intense as it is toward the end of one's training cycle can increase one's likelihood of getting injured, and also of being in a state of energy deficiency.

CONSIDERATIONS

- What are the reasons for holding on to this high-energy load?
- Is this why Jayden has remained injured for so long?
- What would the effect be on performance and healing if exercise intensity and training load were decreased?

Rest: Do I Have To?

For all athletes, rest is important. Athletes looking to get better may falsely think that adding a second training session on the same day will advance their training. According to Renee Urban, PT, board certified in orthopedics, "Many people feel that if they are not reaching their training goals the answer is to train harder. In actuality, they may just need more recovery time." Overtraining may put them more at risk for injury, an energy imbalance (where energy out doesn't match energy in), fatigue, and potentially serious medical complications such as a low heart rate, low blood pressure, or dizziness.

Days off from exercise can help keep a person's energy balance in check. Many athletes say "rest is unnecessary" or is "a waste of time." Often, they perceive rest days as lazy or unproductive. But according to Urban, during exercise the body and muscles undergo stress and strain. "It is essential to allow for adequate recovery, in order to allow the body to return to its optimal state (homeostasis). It is during this time that tissues can heal, energy can be restored, and the body can adapt to be able to handle the stress of exercise next time." Rest helps the muscular, nervous, and immune systems recover, strengthen, and rebuild, while allowing athletes to minimize soreness, inflammation, and illness.

On days off, the body may not technically engage in exercise, but it is very active while healing and repairing itself. These days will help to recharge your batteries and increase your enthusiasm for the sport; after all, doing the same training day after day can be monotonous. Who are you when you are not a dancer? Or a runner? Or a cyclist? You are more than your sport.

What Do You Do on a Rest Day?

Meditation, massage, hot baths, acupuncture, gentle stretching, or yoga can help improve the body's recovery and healing time. Taking naps and resting muscles that are activated during your training is recommended. It will be amazing to see how much power and energy the athlete gets from simply resting. Cross-training, active hot yoga, and cycling do not count as rest days. The idea is to stretch the muscles and let the body heal.

For any person who is recovering from an ED, rest days should be nonnegotiable, and exercise should be contingent on not only being medically cleared but also meeting nutritional needs. Athletes with EDs must be able to adjust their meal plan to account for their activity and be able to sit out when told to do so. They must be able to meet medical and behavioral expectations of their treatment. The scope of the exercise plan and the number of rest days can be determined by the treatment team and might change over time.

Rest Day Nutrition

Eating on rest days can be hard for athletes, and it doesn't help that many have been told to "eat less" or to "avoid carbs" on a rest day. The brain, liver, kidneys, and other parts of the body are working hard and need food for fuel each day regardless of whether or not you moved. Our total energy expenditure consists of a few categories—resting metabolic rate, thermic effect of food (cost of digestion), non-exercise activity thermogenesis (NEAT), and exercise energy expenditure. The resting metabolic rate accounts for approximately 70 to 75 percent of our energy needs. About 10 percent of our energy expenditure is responsible for digestion (thermic effect of food). So whether it's a rest day or a day you are not exercising, the body is busy! Rest days are filled with healing, rebuilding, repairing, and muscle growth and require food, which includes carbohydrates, proteins, fruits/vegetables, fats, and dairy!

Many will feel hungry on rest days and feel confused by it. But it makes perfect sense. The athletes we see in our practice almost always fall short of their nutritional needs on training days. Exercise can suppress hunger. Complicated training schedules and/or logistics may make it difficult to get everything in on training days. We strategically use rest days to catch up on nutrition. While hard for some to do, this is necessary to prevent a low-energy-availability state (which negatively affects performance, hormones, cognitive function, and mood).

When Exercise Needs to Be Shut Down

When someone needs to abstain from exercise, it typically means their body needs time to heal. Even if you are pulled from your main form of exercise, you should carefully consider the total amount of movement that you are doing—up and down the stairs, laundry, shopping, biking around town, and so on. It is important to cut back where possible, especially if you are medically fragile.

Many people struggle with the idea of stopping exercise and eating more. "You want me to sit out of training *and* eat more?" There is an intense fear that without training, one's body will "turn to mush" and that they will only gain fat. However, as a malnourished individual gains weight, they gain in many areas of the body. Weight gain occurs in the muscles, bones, brain, liver, and kidneys. You have read about how several systems in the body shut down due to malnutrition (chapters 2 and 11), and yet with nourishment and weight gain, each of these systems turns back on, thus improving energy, strength, and cognitive function.

As someone heals, and is eventually cleared to return to their sport, it can be challenging for them. This experience can be likened to returning from an injury. We tell our patients to start slowly, at lower intensity and in shorter duration, to help them progress steadily. We often also recommend not jumping into their sport right away but to start with walking, yoga, or stretching and progressing in movement. This helps with training and injury prevention. This is all done while simultaneously monitoring medical status and nutritional needs, and making adjustments as needed. The gradual progression ensures that everything stays in balance along the way.

Allow yourself to consider that your ED was a major assault to the body, affecting every system. It will therefore take time to return to where your athleticism was "before." This would be easy to understand if there had been a physical injury, like an ACL tear.

Returning to your sport will take patience, and initially athletes may be disappointed. "I've lost my strength" or "I can't swim as long" or "My climbing level is so much lower!" This is just temporary! Patients who are now in a better medical and psychological place with a quieter ED come back stronger, faster, and more explosive once their training catches up. Many of our patients started setting personal records and eventually winning national competitions, which they hadn't done even before the ED!

Exercise Avoidance

We've also seen exercise avoidance occur during recovery. This can happen for a variety of reasons. One might be due to body image distress and discomfort in one's new, recovered body. This can make wearing tight exercise clothes or a form-fitting leotard or swimsuit challenging. A person might feel uncomfortable with how it feels to move—the way their thighs rub together during movement, how their stomach looks in a fitted tank top, or how their skin feels on their body from changing body sizes. There might be an avoidance of exercise for fear of being judged, or concern around being teased (due to weight stigma). They may be worried about jeopardizing what they have accomplished during treatment, so they decide they don't want to experiment with altering their meal plan or energy balance to begin activity. They may not feel particularly connected to any one type of activity; perhaps they don't want to go to the gym because it feels forced and isn't fun, but they don't know what else they want to do. Some may feel scarred from a previously unbalanced relationship with exercise; they may feel burned out and may not feel like exercising at this time. They might avoid exercise because they finally found balance, health, and appreciation for their body and are concerned about again becoming compulsive. Or they just don't feel like exercising.

This can be a good time to explore and experiment with different activities that you find most enjoyable. Using an exposure approach can be helpful for those who feel interested but hesitant. With virtual classes, it's easier now to watch a class online and see if it's appealing, or to try out a class in the privacy of your own home. Or you may wish to solidify your recovery for a bit longer before shaking things up.

CHAPTER 14

Pregnancy, Postpartum, and Parenting

THERE ARE MANY nutrition changes and challenges that come with pregnancy, the postpartum period, and parenting.*

There is a lot to cover here, so for ease of reading we will break it down into the following three parts.

1. **Pregnancy:** symptom management, dietary needs, weight gain, and body image

2. **Postpartum:** symptom management, dietary needs, weight loss, and body image

3. **Parenting:** meeting your nutrition needs while caring for children, and modeling food and body positivity to them

No matter where you are on your ED recovery journey, pregnancy can leave you questioning everything. For some, pregnancy is a recovery motivator, for others it's the trigger for developing an ED or a relapse. It's a time of rapid body changes, expected weight gain, and increased nutrient needs. A multitude of symptoms can challenge ED recovery: morning sickness, food aversion, sensitivity to smells, heartburn, and

---

* Please note that this chapter is written about biological females and parts of this chapter may or may not apply to you. Feel free to take what applies and skip what does not.

constipation. Yet staying on track with your nutrition is of the utmost importance for the growth and development of your baby, since insufficient nutrition is associated with miscarriage, stillbirth, and preterm delivery.[1]

There may also be complications that require significant dietary changes, such as gestational diabetes or anemia. Throughout this period, you will want to have close contact with your treatment team to make sure you are adequately supported. From your OB's waiting room to your favorite pregnancy app, you are likely to feel inundated with nutrition information, some of which will be welcome and much of which will be confusing and maybe even maddening. The good news is, there's a tool in your very hands right now that can help (and no, we're not talking about your pregnancy app). The Plate-by-Plate Approach® can provide a huge source of relief during this time, no matter where you are in recovery and your pregnancy. The Plate-by-Plate Approach® was created to provide simplicity throughout your ED recovery journey and beyond. In the following sections of this chapter, we will guide you through general pregnancy nutrition with the help of the Plate-by-Plate Approach®. We will also discuss the challenges that may arise, and we'll provide resources to help you navigate a more specialized diet if needed.

Before You Conceive

As you prepare for pregnancy (if you have the chance to plan) you will want to make sure your body is adequately nourished to support a baby. There is a greater risk for pregnancy complications for women with a history of EDs; these complications include hyperemesis gravidarum (severe nausea and vomiting during pregnancy), spontaneous abortion, and low-birth-weight babies.[2] Poor maternal weight gain and poor nutritional status during pre-pregnancy lead to a smaller placenta, which affects the amount of nutrition the fetus can obtain.[3] Pre-pregnancy nutrition has a consistent connection to infant birth weight. Check in with your doctor beforehand to discuss your health. Are you getting regular periods? If not, is this related to malnutrition? Low weight? Something else entirely?

Amenorrhea and oligomenorrhea are common medical complications resulting from malnutrition, dieting, disordered eating, dysfunctional exercise, bingeing, purging, laxatives, and/or diuretic use and occurs in individuals of all body sizes with EDs. It is important to note, however, that women with amenorrhea can still ovulate and therefore could become pregnant if sexually active. Women with EDs are more likely to have unplanned pregnancies.[4]

Establishing regular periods will be fundamental prior to trying to conceive. Eating regularly, including sufficient dietary fats (helpful for boosting hormones and eventually for the developing baby), including rest days and reducing exercise intensity, managing stress levels, and gaining weight back if needed are helpful strategies to boost hormone levels. These strategies also stimulate metabolism, minimize any existent energy deficiency, and suppress cortisol levels, which affect the hypothalamus and improve reproductive function.

For those undergoing fertility treatments, there can often be quick changes in weight leading to bloating, fatigue, and mood swings. Staying on track with your nutrition plan is important. Using the Plate-by-Plate Approach®, aiming for 3 meals and 2 or 3 snacks per day including all 5 food groups at meals and at least 2 or 3 different food groups at snacks, will help you meet your baseline needs. In addition, if you haven't already, you will want to start taking a prenatal supplement that ideally includes iron, folate, and DHA to help fill any nutritional gaps and meet the increased vitamin and mineral requirements of pregnancy. It's important to note that although taking prenatal supplements is commonly recommended by medical and nutrition professionals, they're not meant to replace food.

Prenatal vitamins should be started *prior to* trying to conceive. Getting in 400 mg a day of folate is especially important to prevent neural tube defects as seen in spina bifida. Folic acid is found in leafy, dark green vegetables (e.g., spinach), citrus fruits, nuts, legumes, whole grains, and fortified bread and cereals, though it has been found that getting in enough folate from food alone is often difficult.[5] Low iron can affect fetal brain structure, and low zinc can affect neural tube closures. Adequate vitamin and mineral status and good overall health before pregnancy is strongly linked to favorable pregnancy outcomes.[6]

Changes in Body: Weight Gain

Weight gain and body changes are necessary in pregnancy to ensure the health of your baby. Weight gain will be used to support all aspects of the pregnancy, from the growing baby (including the placenta and amniotic fluid) to the mother (maternal tissues needed to support the pregnancy, extra blood volume, fluids, uterus, mammary glands, and fat stores).[7] This can be challenging for those in ED recovery.

Some might have just become used to their recovered body that enabled them to even get pregnant, and now they face having to get used to a new body. Others might have never even been comfortable in their body to begin with. Many express concerns. *What will this feel like? What will my body be like afterward? What will it feel like if I can't exercise as much?* Pregnancy is an adventure, and the start of an even bigger adventure to come: motherhood. Surrendering your body to the growing baby inside is just the beginning of the sacrifices that a mother makes for her child.

We have had patients use their pregnancy as a powerful recovery motivator, abandoning their ED to provide the fullest possible nutrition to their growing baby. This has been amazing to watch. They have shared their joy about their increasing hormones, expanding belly, and weight gain, and have even loved eating more full meals and snacks.

All pregnant individuals will be expected to gain weight during this time to support their pregnancy. Failure to gain weight or gain enough weight is a red flag and should be addressed with your health provider. The body will change shape during pregnancy. Fat is stored in different parts of the body, all with the same purpose: to nourish and protect your growing baby. The following weight gain recommendations are from the CDC,[8] but no weight gain guidelines have been established for extremely low pre-pregnancy weights, so these guidelines should be individualized.[9]

Weight Gain Recommendations during Pregnancy

PRE-PREGNANCY BMI	RECOMMENDED WEIGHT GAIN DURING PREGNANCY ONE BABY (POUNDS)	RECOMMENDED WEIGHT GAIN DURING PREGNANCY TWINS (POUNDS)
<18.5	28–40	50–62
18.5–24.9	25–35	37–54
25.0–29.9	15–25	31–50
30.0 +	11–20	24–42

Your doctor will weigh you at each prenatal appointment to be sure you are on track. If hearing or tracking your weight is triggering, anxiety-producing, or just not helpful in your recovery process and pregnancy, consider speaking to your medical team about taking blind weights at each appointment (so your doctor can track your weight gain without your seeing it). Many ob-gyns are not trained in ED management and might not be versed at practicing weight-inclusive care. Be sure to chat with them about your expectations for care. It might sound something like this:

"I don't want to see the number on the scale. Please inform the support staff as well, so they don't accidentally leave my weight record in the exam room. This would be very triggering for me."

"I have a history of an eating disorder."

"Please don't comment about my food intake."

"Please don't comment about my weight unless you have a concern about which I need to be aware, and even then, please inform me of the concern—and not the number."

Then your doctor can talk to you about trends instead of exact numbers, which may be more helpful in your recovery process. If your experience with weight gain and the ever-changing shape of your body is difficult to process, please speak with your team about how to manage this distress and check out our helpful tips in chapter 18. A healthy baby needs a healthy mama; the work you do now will assure you and your baby a successful pregnancy and postpartum journey together.

Nutritional Needs in Pregnancy

Nutrition needs change considerably during pregnancy. Because of this, there is a seemingly endless supply of dos and don'ts that can cause anyone with an ED to feel restricted at a time when they need to feel flexible with food. While there are a few very important don'ts to adhere to in pregnancy—including alcohol, caffeine, seafood, undercooked meat or eggs, and unpasteurized foods—most recommendations are not so absolute.

Changing Nutrition Needs in Pregnancy

Your baseline needs will remain largely unchanged in the first trimester and will increase by the beginning of your second trimester.[10] By the second trimester, the amount of the increase depends on the individual, but it's commonly estimated that for an otherwise healthy person, nutrition needs will increase by about the equivalent of one 3-item snack per day (e.g., yogurt + granola + berries). By the third trimester, that amount increases by another additional food item (yogurt + granola + berries + almonds). That amount stays consistent in the postpartum period for those who choose to breastfeed.

Protein needs increase during pregnancy, but if you are following the Plate-by-Plate Approach®, this difference is minor (see page 196). Pregnancy will be accompanied by an increase in aversions to food. This can make it hard for women to meet their protein requirements, so it might mean adding new, previously unexplored sources like dairy (kefir, cottage cheese, cheese, yogurt) or nuts, beans, or tofu, or adding protein bars or protein-rich smoothies. Those in larger bodies with higher needs overall might need to add a second protein serving to their plates to ensure they get enough at their meals. For further customization, consult with a registered dietitian.

Recommended Daily Allowance for Protein Needs*

STAGE	DAILY ALLOWANCE
Pre-pregnancy	0.8 g/kg
Pregnancy	1.1 g/kg
Lactation (0–6 months post-delivery)	1.1 g/kg

To calculate weight into kilograms, divide your weight in pounds by 2.2.

*All this is assuming your nutrition is adequate prior to conception.

Energy and Fluid Requirements During and After Pregnancy*

STAGE	NUTRITION RECOMMENDATIONS	FLUIDS
First Trimester	No change	
Second Trimester	Add the equivalent of a 3-item snack	8–12 cups or 64–96 oz fluids*
Third Trimester	Add the equivalent of a 4-item snack	8–12 cups or 64–96 oz fluids*
Lactation	Add the equivalent of a 4-item snack	16 cups or 128 oz fluids per day
Postpartum Needs (non-lactating)	Similar to your pre-pregnancy baseline needs: 3 meals + 2–3 snacks per day)	See fluid guidelines on pages 41–43

*Can come from food and beverages[11]

For those in need of weight gain prior to pregnancy, you'll want to work closely with your team to be sure you are able to eat enough to meet your nutritional goals. This will likely look similar to the Accelerated Plate (see chapter 6 for ideas on ways to increase your meals and snacks). You may need to add beverages to meals or to have larger or more frequent snacks to gain the weight needed to support a healthy pregnancy. Eating 3 full meals (including all 5 food groups) and 2 or 3 (or more) snacks per day, and choosing from a variety of different food groups, will provide your body with adequate nutrition. Taking a daily prenatal supplement will help fill any vitamin and mineral gaps but does not replace food!

While not all micronutrient needs increase during pregnancy, many do. Below is a table of the recommended dietary allowances (RDA) of several vitamins and minerals for pregnant and lactating women, which highlights those differences. Except for calcium, most of these vitamins and minerals are found in prenatal supplements (calcium is the exception due to its large molecular size and is more commonly consumed through calcium-rich foods and separate calcium supplements).

Recommended Dietary Allowances During Pregnancy and Lactation[12]

NUTRIENT (MG/D*)	PREGNANT**	LACTATION**
Vitamin A	770	1,300
Vitamin D	15	15
Vitamin E	15	19
Vitamin K	90	90
Folate	600	500
Niacin	18	17
Riboflavin	1.4	1.6
Thiamin	1.4	1.4
Vitamin B_6	1.9	2
Vitamin B_{12}	2.6	2.8
Vitamin C	85	120
Calcium	1,000	1,000
Iron	27	9
Phosphorus	700	700
Selenium	60	70
Zinc	11	12

*Milligrams per deciliter
**For women age 18+

Orthorexia in Pregnancy

Beyond the well-established dos and don'ts, there is a lot of gray area. It's not uncommon to start fearing anything you put in your body. What if your produce isn't organic? Are the crackers you keep at your bedside to combat nausea too processed? Are the lime Popsicles you crave multiple times each day going to give you gestational diabetes? The list of "what ifs" can seem endless, and with Google at your fingertips, it's easy to see why those in treatment for EDs while pregnant are at high risk for developing orthorexia.

Other than the list of "don'ts," just about all food is free to eat and explore. Some recommendations are helpful but not required. For example, there are some studies about pesticide exposure in pregnancy. If you can't even stomach the smell of broccoli during your first trimester, why bother worrying if your produce is organic or not? Perhaps you're on a tight budget and conventional produce is what's affordable and available—it's certainly better to include thoroughly washed, nonorganic fruits and veggies than to avoid produce completely.

Your health is vital to the growth and development of your baby. If you have become so restrictive and limited in what you will and will not eat, you might not be eating enough. This can affect your ability to stay on track with weight expectations, which could in turn affect fetal growth. Thinking or obsessing about food intake can increase your stress levels and cause you to withdraw socially, too—all of which can increase anxiety and depression. Liberalizing your diet can add more nutrients, expand access to foods, and help you meet your needs during this important time. If you feel plagued by anxiety related to how "clean" your food is, please refer to chapter 15 for tips on food exposure to challenge ED thinking and expand your variety (at least as soon as your nausea and food aversions subside).

Common Pregnancy Symptoms (with Nutritional Implications)

Though each individual will experience pregnancy differently, several symptoms are commonly encountered. We will cover the symptoms with nutritional implications here.

Nausea

Nausea (with or without vomiting) is commonly referred to as morning sickness. For women of all sizes, persistent nausea and vomiting can have serious medical consequences, including dehydration, electrolyte imbalances, and/or weight loss, and this has been the leading cause of first-trimester hospital admissions.[13]

Tips for combating nausea during pregnancy

- In case nausea strikes first thing in the morning, keep a snack next to your bed to eat before you even fully wake up (e.g., crackers, nuts, dried fruit).

- If eating 3 larger meals and 2 or 3 snacks per day doesn't help, try eating 6 evenly sized small meals throughout the day.

- If food odors are a problem, ask a loved one to cook for you and leave the room while they are cooking.

- Stay hydrated throughout the day by taking frequent sips of hot or cold liquids.

- Take prenatal supplements *with* food.

- Ginger has known anti-nausea properties,[14] so try ginger tea or ginger chews.

- Try limiting spicy foods if they bother you.

- Use of essential oils (lavender or mint) can be helpful.

- Open windows to circulate fresh air and keep room temperatures mild.

See tips on nausea in chapter 9. If these tips don't help, please discuss your symptoms further with your health care provider.

Food cravings

Food cravings and aversions are another common symptom during pregnancy, and there are many theories about why they occur. One is that aversions prevent the mother from eating foods that may be harmful to the baby, and cravings increase the intake of foods needed for the baby's growth. With that said, there are very few foods that can cause actual harm to a growing baby in our modern world. It can be valuable to lean into your cravings while you try to incorporate a wide variety of food groups throughout the day.

Cravings may be driven by nutritional needs and might help you meet your unique needs during pregnancy. They can also be a confusing symptom for those in ED recovery. Leaning into food cravings requires some level of food intuition. If you are just beginning your recovery, you are likely not yet eating intuitively. In this case, sticking with 3 meals (including all 5 food groups) and 2 or 3 snacks (of 2 or 3 food groups each) per day will allow you to get the nutrition you need for you and baby, while supporting your ED recovery goals. If you are unable to meet your nutrition goals using this approach, we strongly recommend discussing a more personalized plan with your treatment team.

Heartburn

Are you struggling with heartburn, otherwise known as acid reflux? Hormones cause relaxation of the esophageal sphincter, a ring of muscle that opens and closes to allow food into the stomach. Its primary job is to ensure that food and stomach acids stay in the stomach and do not back up into the esophagus. Increasing levels of progesterone during pregnancy slows the digestive process, keeping food in the stomach for a longer period of time, which can contribute to acid reflux. Later in pregnancy, the upward pressure of the growing uterus also contributes to acid reflux.[15] Antacids may be a common remedy for acid reflux, but the truth is that the acid in your stomach is beneficial. It kills harmful bacteria, digests protein, and absorbs vitamin B$_{12}$. By decreasing the acid in your stomach, you run the risk of food poisoning, digestive problems, and nutrient deficiencies. Plus, some heartburn is a result of too little acid, not too much.[16]

Tips for managing heartburn

- Try eating 6 similarly sized meals rather than 3 meals and 2 or 3 snacks per day so that the quantity of food you consume at any given time is consistent and smaller than a typical meal but adequate to meet your daily needs.

- Consider drinking water and other beverages between meals rather than with meals.

- Limit late-night eating so that you have time to digest your food before lying down to sleep (which can exacerbate heartburn). If you need a snack before bed, consider something that's easy to digest such as plain crackers or a banana.

- Minimize caffeine intake.

- Opt for nonacidic fruits and fruit juices such as banana, apple, mango, and melon.

- Limit spicy food.

- Swap non-carbonated water and other beverages for the carbonated variety.

- Try ginger tea or chews to combat reflux.

- If you love herbal tea, chamomile is a great choice over mint (which tends to worsen reflux).

- Tomatoes and foods with tomato sauce are known to exacerbate reflux.

- Sleeping upright on an incline can help.[17]

Constipation and hemorrhoids

Constipation is thought to be caused by hormonal shifts beginning in the first trimester and including physical changes of the body as the uterus grows to make space for your growing baby during the second and third trimesters. Increased progesterone levels slow bowel motility, leading to constipation in some pregnant individuals. Slowed motility allows the body to absorb more water and nutrients for mom and baby. Unfortunately, this can cause stool to be dry and hard to pass.

Additionally, the weight of the fetus and the pressure on the veins leads to the development of hemorrhoids. Along with hormone shifts, prenatal supplements (specifically those containing iron) may be to blame. To manage this unfavorable symptom of pregnancy, the following tips may be helpful.

1.   Increase fluids (water, juice, milk, Popsicles, soup).

2.   Increase fiber-containing foods (fruits and veggies, whole grains, beans, and nuts). Be careful not to overdo it, as too much fiber can worsen constipation, gas, and bloating. A good rule of thumb is to increase your baseline fiber content slowly to allow your body to get used to this dietary change. Small changes such as adding in a few prunes each day can help. Increasing fluids at the same time as increasing fiber will help your body tolerate this change.

3.   Physical activity helps prevent constipation. Make sure to check with your medical provider about what type of physical activity is safe for you during your pregnancy.

Fatigue

Fatigue is a common and often overwhelming symptom of pregnancy, particularly in the first and third trimesters. In the first trimester, hormonal changes are thought to be the cause as the body boosts blood flow to the uterus. In the third trimester, increased physical discomfort and disrupted sleep are more likely to be the cause of fatigue. Either way, here are a few ways that you can manage your fatigue.

1.   Maintain blood sugar levels by eating 3 meals (including all 5 food groups) and 2 or 3 snacks (including 2 or 3 different items) each day.

2.   Stay hydrated.

3.   Take a daily prenatal vitamin.

4.   Stay physically active (consult with your medical provider about what type and amount of physical activity is safe for you during your pregnancy).

5.   Don't hesitate to take a nap. For some of you, this will be a new experience. Listen to your body.

6. Check in with your doctor to be sure you are making expected gains to support your pregnancy, and that your labs are within normal limits (iron levels can drop during pregnancy, causing fatigue). Ask for an assesssment of other potential medical causes for fatigue.

Gestational diabetes

Throughout your pregnancy, your medical provider will be checking regular blood work and will likely require you to take a glucose toler-ance test to check for signs of gestational diabetes. Gestational diabetes occurs when the mother's body has difficulty using or making enough insulin.[18] This leads to high blood sugar levels, which can impact both the mother's and the baby's health. This can be a hard diagnosis for many, and especially hard for those with either a history of ED or an active ED who have been working hard to rebuild their relationship with food. Some might wonder, "Did my recovery cause this?" No! "Do I now have to diet?" Definitely not!

The good news is that gestational diabetes is highly treatable through dietary changes, exercise, and blood glucose monitoring. The bad news is that it can pose particular challenges for individuals with EDs because it may increase your preoccupation with and attention to food. Of course, this diagnosis also causes a lot of worry for expectant mothers. It might be tempting to restrict foods, but dieting isn't the answer. Dieting might increase the risk for bingeing, purging, or lax-ative use, which can make controlling your blood sugar even more dif-ficult, while increasing your medical risk of electrolyte abnormalities. Keeping up with expected weight gain is necessary for the growth and development of your baby, so weight loss is not recommended. Regular medical visits will be necessary to check on your health and the baby's. Speak to your team about ways to carefully alter your diet and activity level while also protecting your recovery. You can continue to utilize the Plate-by-Plate Approach®[19] and your dietitian can help you make man-ageable changes to lower your blood sugar levels.

Preeclampsia

Preeclampsia is a type of hypertension (high blood pressure) that occurs during pregnancy. If left untreated, preeclampsia can lead to serious, life-threatening consequences for mom and baby. Symptoms may include protein in the urine, kidney damage, preterm labor, decreased platelets, elevated liver enzymes, headaches, dizziness, blurred visions, nausea, and edema (swelling). This can be stressful, but it's important to stay on track with regular meals to stay nourished. Contrary to what you may have heard about the role of dietary salt on blood pressure, a low-sodium diet is not recommended during pregnancy, mostly because it has not been shown to be effective.[20] Staying hydrated, staying active, and consuming adequate protein can help. Please check with your doctor for more individualized dietary guidance to help manage preeclampsia.

Exercise

Women who have no contraindications to exercise and have been assessed by their medical doctor are generally considered cleared to exercise while pregnant. Monitoring should be continually assessed by one's doctor. Moving during pregnancy is associated with many benefits, such as higher likelihood of vaginal delivery; lower risk of hypertensive disorders, gestational diabetes, preterm birth, and low birth weight; and less depression postpartum.[21] However, it's important to note that too much exercise can be concerning. In a case-control study of 526 women, those who exercised more than 5 times per week while pregnant were 4.6 times more likely to give birth to a low-for-gestational-weight baby.[22] In addition, exercising beyond 45 minutes at high intensities when pregnant can lead to hypoglycemia (low blood sugar). Therefore, it is recommended to ensure adequate nutrition before training, and/or limiting duration and intensity as necessary.[23]

High-impact sports—or any activities in which there is risk of blunt trauma to the mother or fetus—should be avoided. Monitoring for hyperthermia, electrolytes, hydration, energy balance, and expected weight gain are all important factors to consider. It is important to work closely with your team to meet nutritional needs and to ensure a healthy pregnancy outcome.

You should stop exercising immediately if you experience head-aches, dizziness, shortness of breath, vaginal bleeding, abdominal pain, amniotic fluid leakage, chest pain, painful contractions, muscle weakness affecting balance, or calf pain or swelling.[24]

Postpartum

During this stage, there's a lot of "newness" to adjust to—every day. Motherhood is an incredible ride! Your body will not feel like your own after having a baby. It's different, and trying to get your "pre-baby body" back is an irrational goal that only exists to make you feel like a failure.

The reality is, you can't get your "pre-baby body" back because you had a baby. Your body will forever be a "post-baby body" and that's great! What an absolute miracle you just made happen! You grew a human inside your body, and that is an accomplishment you can carry with you for the rest of your life. To reiterate: You grew a human inside your body! If that statement makes you feel proud, and then five seconds later you feel sad about the loss of your "pre-baby body," that's normal and okay. This postpartum period is all about adjusting to new norms and seeking the support you need to do so.

Immediately after having a baby, you will still look pregnant (but with a jelly-like belly because the baby is no longer inside you). You will also likely have most of the weight you gained during pregnancy still on your body (minus the weight of the baby, as well as bodily fluids lost during labor and delivery). It took about 40 weeks to gain the weight needed to support a healthy baby during pregnancy and it will take just as long (or maybe longer) for the body to readjust. For individuals who were underweight prior to pregnancy, retaining some of that pregnancy weight may be necessary to maintain optimal health postpartum. For others, weight might return to somewhere in the ballpark of what it was pre-pregnancy but the body shape is different. Perhaps your hips are wider, your breasts are larger (or higher or lower), you may be los-ing hair or growing hair, you may smell differently, you have stretch marks in many new places, you might have larger or wider feet, your skin might feel looser, and you might feel wobbly and jiggly. If reading all this makes you feel uncomfortable, sad, frustrated, angry, anxious, or depressed, please call on your support system to help you process it. You will need their support to grieve the loss of your "pre-baby body" and embrace your current, life-giving body so that you can enjoy this time with the baby that you nurtured and grew.

Nutrition needs won't differ a whole lot during the postpartum period compared to the third trimester of pregnancy (especially if you are choosing to breastfeed). You should continue to eat 3 meals and 2 or 3 (or more!) snacks per day that include all the food groups. You should also continue taking your prenatal vitamins for at least six months postpartum or if and for as long as you're breastfeeding. It's important to replenish the nutrients lost from pregnancy and delivery and to support the increased needs of lactation. After you give birth, a natural slowing down happens. It can feel hard to ask for help, but allow others to care for and feed you so that you can feed and care for your newborn.

If you choose to breastfeed, you will need to consider extra hydration (from a variety of fluids, including water) and extra food. Breastfeeding is nutritionally demanding, and you will need to keep up with your energy and fluid needs in order to build and then maintain your milk supply. Keep a very large bottle or jug nearby at all times. It's easiest if it contains a straw so you can sip on it throughout the day. Nursing women require about 16 cups (128 ounces) of fluids each day to support lactation. It can come from food, beverages, and water.[25] A good rule of thumb is to drink fluids anytime your baby is nursing.

As always, if you have any questions about the safety of your diet while breastfeeding or are struggling to keep up with the nutritional demands of breastfeeding, please consult your treatment team.

Perinatal Mood and Anxiety Disorders

Untreated anxiety or depression will greatly affect your ability to nourish yourself sufficiently. An insufficient amount of food and fluids can have a negative effect on breast milk production. This can also affect the energy required to care for your newborn, as well as your medical status (vital signs, hormones, metabolism, and recovery from childbirth).

Stress management and getting enough rest, nutrition, time off, and hydration are some of the self-care tools every new mother needs to help ease the transition into motherhood.

Parenting

Eating 3 meals and 2 or 3 snacks per day can feel like an impossible task to accomplish when you are caring for children. Whether you have a newborn who needs 24-7 care or a fourteen-year-old who needs to be chauffeured to various after-school engagements, it can be challenging to take time to nourish yourself. But your needs are every bit as important as your children's. They depend on you and need you to be healthy. They're also watching what and how you eat, which can create an enormous amount of pressure for you to recover (for better or worse.)

It can be helpful to tell yourself, "When they eat, I eat." If you are making breakfast each morning for your children but skipping it yourself, that's an opportunity to eat. Make yourself breakfast while you're making it for your children and sit down with them to eat it. If you are packing lunches for your kids to bring to school, pack one for yourself to take to work. If you stay home with your children, make lunch for all of you to eat together. When you serve your children snacks at home, in the car, at the playground or soccer field, make extras for yourself!

Family meals have been shown to increase a child's social competencies and help foster positive identity. Research shows that regular family meals improve physical, social-emotional, and academic benefits. Conversely, fewer family meals have been shown to contribute to a child's high-risk behaviors, such as substance use, sexual activity, suicide, antisocial behaviors, violence, school problems, binge eating, purging, and excessive weight loss.[26]

If eating with your children is a struggle and you're worried about the impact that may have on their relationship with food, consider asking your partner, family member, or friend to eat with your children until you are able to do so. You can also consider asking a partner or loved one to do food preparation so that you can focus solely on eating. If you're a new parent and can't find the time to eat, let alone cook a meal, ask for support. You may need to buy pre-made meals for a while or rely on family, friends, and neighbors to bring ready-made meals on a regular basis until you have more time and motivation. And of course, if your growing family is causing financial strain and you're finding it difficult to afford food, please see Resources, page 304.

Raising Body-Positive Kids and Teens

Parents are often concerned about how they can raise confident eaters with positive body image if they themselves are struggling. A British study found that 15.3 percent of women will have had an ED before their first pregnancy.[27] Tips for creating a body-positive household include the following.[28]

1. **Avoid polarization of foods.** Polarizing foods ("good" and "bad" foods) disconnects us from our body's true wisdom and often indirectly reinforces messaging about dieting and losing weight. Talking about "fattening foods" is scientifically untrue—it is scientifically incorrect that fat in food makes you fat—and it teaches kids to fear and loathe fatness (fatphobia). Any one food does not have the power to cause weight gain. This language teaches children to fear ostensibly bad foods and tiptoe around eating. It sends the indirect message that being fat is bad and being thin is good.

2. **Avoid exercising to burn calories, lose weight, or alter one's appearance.** This creates an unhealthy relationship with physical activity. Linking exercise to food intake in any way ("I ate so much today, so I'm going to exercise") teaches kids that they should compensate with exercise for food consumed, which is a dangerous and disturbing message, and over time can lead to the development of an ED. Parents can emphasize the many wonderful benefits of exercise, such as stress relief and an improvement in mood, energy, and sleep. It is well documented that individuals who exercise for internal goals, camaraderie, energy, or stress relief are more likely to continue their habit of moving than those who exercise based on external goals such as the pursuit of thinness.

3. **Create a judgment-free zone.** This zone is also free of get-thin messages, allowing kids to grow up more peacefully with their

body regardless of its size. This is especially important during adolescence, when kids may feel uncomfortable and confused by their changing bodies. In households where parents commented on their children's bodies, those children were more likely to engage in binge eating, secretive eating, or disordered eating.[29]

4. **Make home a place of safety.** Home should be free of conversation about how your child's body looks or should look, how you look, how your clothes fit, or how others look. Avoid thin-biases. Teach kids that all bodies are good bodies, and that if their body is bigger or smaller or changing sizes in any way, you will love them no matter what.

5. **Avoid commenting on people's bodies.** When parents talk at the dinner table and comment about people's weight—"Did you see so-and-so? He/she/they looks great!"—they automatically glamorize thinness through perceived signaling that thinness is idealized and valued, and if children want to be praised and adored, she/he/they "should be" thin. Even saying things such as "No, that does not make you look fat," stigmatizes fat, suggesting there is something wrong with a higher weight.

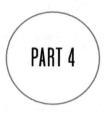

PART 4

Food Freedom

CHAPTER 15

Moving Beyond Food Fears

THE JOURNEY OF ED recovery continues even after one restores weight, stabilizes vital signs and metabolism, and even normalizes hormones. As some of you arrive at this point, you may wish to be "done," to close this chapter of your recovery. You may also know deep down that you need more help before you can be fully present in your life. *Food fears* are lingering, gnawing, stealing their presence and attention.

Food fear is an irrational belief that certain foods are going to harm you in some way. There is usually an escalation of anxiety when presented with these foods or in certain situations around food. The anxiety varies in degree, ranging from mild to extremely intense. The specific feared foods, rules, or food situations vary by person and may be left over from something the ED latched on to—a comment from a parent, a friend, a coach, or something you read. Many have told us they have no idea why they follow certain rules or avoid certain items. The more that foods are avoided, the scarier they become.

These fears have likely held you back in some way. We have heard heartbreaking stories of people missing out on pivotal life events such as family celebrations, vacations, birthday meals, and holidays. Individuals with avoidant/restrictive food intake disorder (ARFID) might have aversions to textures, smells, or certain types of foods and can use these same principles of food exposure and desensitization. They might have a strong reaction (nausea or gagging) to certain foods.

Those with limited preferences can use the principles of food exposure to expand their preferences if they're ready and if the exposures are unpressured and collaborative. Those who struggle with binge eating may be more likely to binge on foods they avoid. You crave that which you forbid!

A focus of exposure work for those who binge is to allow foods that have been excluded. This might need to be done slowly, gradually, with supervision or with the assistance of a partner, or out of the house to start—by going out for ice cream or having dessert at a friend's house, for example.

Many of our neurodivergent patients rely on the same foods each day for stability and safety. In this case, a person might work on rotating foods among a list of preferred foods that feel safe. Those who are neurodiverse might find too many foods or colors on a plate overstimulating, and might come to rely on foods with certain textures, tastes, and smells. If change happens, it might be slow. One of our patients with AN and autism spectrum disorder (ASD) shared, "I think people with ASD change at a much slower pace and require time to adapt, so an exposure might take two or three times as long. But that doesn't mean it isn't worth it."

Do you have vivid memories of being forced by a parent or treatment center to do an exposure when you were younger? These historical exposures often come with mixed feelings: resentment, anger, frustration, and maybe a tiny bit of relief, because many knew they couldn't and wouldn't do the exposures on their own. But now, as adults, you get to decide how this part of your journey will look or whether you will begin at all.

Throughout this chapter, we will uncover what food fears still exist for you. You will be your own detective and discover more about your food rules and the ways the ED might still be breathing beneath the surface—perhaps holding you back from eating in restaurants or going out with friends.

Food Freedom

Food freedom is the power to make food choices without any hindrance or restraint. It's the idea of eating freely and calmly, while embracing all foods.

What might it be like for you to be free?

What are your goals?

How do you envision your recovery?

Is this something you want to work toward?

Be Your Own Detective

Imagine joyfully eating birthday cake without fear, choosing what you really want from the restaurant menu, or grabbing pizza with friends without hesitating. Imagine saying yes to a dinner date or travel plans without worrying about how to "manage" the food. Flexibility and food variety are essential for becoming open to and accepting of all foods, which ultimately helps eliminate food anxiety.

Living fully and freely requires you to be a good detective, to evaluate all the ways the ED might be subconsciously lurking. We want you to be on the lookout for remnants of the ED. We will ask you which foods escalate anxiety and whether there are still rules that you might not have even realized you are still following. Here is an example.

> Stace shared they weren't comfortable having dessert in the afternoon. Their ED had created this idea that dessert "had to be" eaten only in the evening. They challenged this idea in treatment and were surprised to see that "nothing happened" when they had dessert one Wednesday afternoon. This enabled Stace to grab ice cream with friends or say yes to afternoon desserts at work, which finally meant they could actually participate in celebrating their colleague's birthday.

Returning to baseline

What did you love before the ED took hold? What were your favorite meals? Favorite snacks? Restaurants? Are those old favorites part of your life now? If not, why not? Before the ED developed, there might have been an ease, a joy, and a spontaneity around food. Perhaps those food experiences are something you can revisit as you explore and investigate your current relationship with food.

On the other hand, we have heard some people share, "I hated how I used to eat, that's why I developed an eating disorder." Perhaps "before" there were chaotic nutritional habits, frequently skipped meals, grazing without structure, or structure without spontaneity. Or maybe you just generally disliked food back then so you didn't pay much attention. Maybe going "exactly back to how it was" doesn't feel quite right, but staying here doesn't feel quite right either. Maybe you can find a middle ground or reprise some aspects of your old way of eating. For example, perhaps you like how you used to be flexible and spontaneous and never worried about food or cared whether the meal timing was off.

Eating in community, and with family

Being able to share meals with loved ones is an important aspect of food, culture, celebration, and religion. Eating together is an important part of many cultural experiences, such as holiday meals. Eating with others can be a time to unwind, to set aside chores, obligations, and the stresses of the day. This can provide support, boundaries, and accountability and can reinforce one's commitment to recovery. When you cook or dine with others, meals are likelier to contain more food groups and be more creative and inventive, which can be beneficial for your ED in the long run.

For many people with EDs, eating with others can be stressful. Conversation, social dynamics, new foods, and the fear of people watching you can be intimidating. Eating in a group setting can be especially difficult for those with social anxiety or ASD or for those who have difficulty making eye contact or starting conversations. With ASD patients, social settings can also be overstimulating and loud, adding to the difficult environment.

How do you feel about eating with others? For some, it might be easier to eat with one's inner circle, like parents, children, or a loved one. And some might find it hard to eat with their extended circle, like friends or coworkers. Some find it easier or harder to eat with strangers.

Do you feel better with some distraction? Some of our patients prefer to listen to music or wear earplugs while eating in a crowded environment or to watch a show on their phone while eating. While this is not "social," it might be the best they can do if they "have to" be in a circumstance that pushes them out of their comfort zone.

Are you able to participate in a family or community meal? Can you join in what your friends and family have chosen to eat, or can you work toward this? If not, consider adding this as a goal in your list of exposures at the end of this chapter.

Ditching dietary restrictions

If you are gluten-free, dairy-free, sugar-free, or fructose-free, finding foods to eat when away from your home environment can be difficult. The more limitations, the greater the challenges. Eating out, traveling, and visiting friends' houses is challenging for those with food allergies/intolerances, and often they need to bring their own food with them to ensure safety. The medical complications are serious and real, and avoiding these foods is a must for many people.

And yet (you knew this was coming) for many people with EDs, there might be "extra" or "lingering" exclusions. An extra exclusion is something someone might have tried omitting as an experiment to heal an ailment like a stomachache, migraine, or fatigue. Even once they realized it didn't provide relief, they never added it back to their diet. An extra exclusion can also be something that their ED thought was "a good idea to cut out"—meaning, it's a vehicle to "restrict more" or to "help them to lose weight." Their diet is left very narrow, and they end up with long lists of foods to avoid and barely remember why they eliminated these foods in the first place.

The goal is full expansion of foods you can eat to be free, to travel, and to participate more fully in life. We ask you, is there something you are avoiding currently that you don't *need* to be avoiding? Is there something you could try again? Of course, only you can answer this. The answer might be no, you cannot change anything. And that's okay. This section might be hard for those who desperately long for more freedom but simply can't achieve the freedom they want because of their intolerances. So many people *want to* try eliminated foods again but are bound to what their bodies will allow. We see you.

For those of you who might be able to add something back into your diet that you haven't had for a while, it might be a catch-22. For example, the body needs dairy to stimulate the production of lactase enzymes. So you will have to eat dairy for the body to make those enzymes to help aid digestion. It can take some time before you can easily tolerate dairy again. Gluten can take some time, too. But a gradual reintroduction is worth the expanded options you will have!

Letting go of being vegetarian or vegan

As with diet restrictions, we often see a switch to vegetarianism just as the ED began. Sometimes the ED and vegetarianism arrive together genuinely, as people begin to learn more about food, cooking, and nutrition. But sometimes, the ED is looking for another way to exclude an additional food category. Vegetarianism that starts when an ED begins feels different from vegetarianism in someone who was, for example, born into a vegetarian family or someone whose vegetarianism predated the ED by many years. When the ED and vegetarianism emerge simultaneously, it's more likely that the reasons for becoming a vegetarian are driven by the ED. We ask you to consider the following.

- When did you become a vegetarian/vegan and when did the ED begin? Did vegetarianism/veganism begin for animal-rights reasons many years before the onset of the ED? Did your ED and vegetarianism begin concurrently? Timing is critical: The closer the start of the vegetarianism is to the onset of the ED, the higher the likelihood that the vegetarianism is *part* of the ED.

- Did you turn to vegetarianism/veganism on a whim? Maybe because you thought it seemed interesting after watching a documentary or because a friend or relative was experimenting with it?

- Did you turn to vegetarianism/veganism because it aligns wholeheartedly with your core beliefs about animal rights, climate change, and/or the environment? Or did it start as an attempt to reduce or alter calories or as a vehicle to diet?

- Are you eating a certain way because a parent or partner ate/eats that way, or because you have been encouraged by your doctor to eat a certain way because of a medical condition? Is this way of eating right *for you*?

- Does this way of eating make you feel good? Or does it reinforce your food fears?

Consider when and how your current food restrictions emerged. If eating in a certain way aligns with your core beliefs, okay. If it emerged on a whim *and* is getting in the way of your ability to be successful, you might want to reevaluate your stance. Changing food behaviors, especially when they are more restrictive, can hold back your progress in recovery. Find other ways to be more environmentally friendly that don't limit your food options, like taking public transportation, composting, and recycling. If you are in need of change, perhaps you can change your hair color! Or your wardrobe! But heed caution with respect to cutting out foods.

If it's difficult to tease out what emerged first, the food restriction or the ED, we encourage you to consider adding those restricted foods back to your diet until you have recovered from your ED. Otherwise, you may be inadvertently keeping that ED alive. Ask yourself: What does my recovery-self need now? Only you know what is in your heart and what is going to be part of your future. Any decision in which the ED is in the driver's seat is most likely not a decision that is aligned with recovery.

With that in mind, is being vegetarian or vegan something that you wish to hang on to in the future? And if it is, are you eating in the most expansive way possible? You can still follow the Plate-by-Plate Approach®, filling up the plate with all food groups to ensure it's enough.

It is still possible to hide behind being vegetarian or vegan to remain restrictive, thereby keeping the ED alive.

If you're struggling, you might use being vegetarian or vegan to get out of eating certain side dishes or even entire meals. For example, at a barbecue you might end up just taking salad and skipping most of the meal that night. A restrictive mindset might be, "Oh well, there was nothing for me to eat." Someone who was more recovery-minded might bring veggie burgers to throw on the grill, anticipating that there could be limited options, or would make up for the lack of plant-based protein sources by filling their plate with sides. Or if there weren't enough options, they would make up for the inadequate meal by eating more when they got home.

Is there too much focus on safe, "clean" foods?

We often hear our patients say that they "don't like" white rice, or just "don't like pancakes." But who is it really that doesn't like these foods . . . you or your ED? Many of these same patients are overly focused on whole grains, unprocessed foods, and avoiding white flour and sugar. One client shared, "Whole grains are healthier, so why *ever* have white bread? It's a waste of calories." But all foods provide energy and nutrients, even white rice and white bread. Your body benefits from variety, so being able to eat flexibly is important.

A varied diet will also ensure that an individual is meeting their fiber needs. For example, beans, cereals, fruits, and vegetables all contain fiber. Physiologically, white and wheat grains are broken down in the body in a similar way. The body uses and digests them similarly, breaking them both down to glucose. We see people obsess about eating brown rice versus white rice, but it is a myth that brown rice is healthier than white rice. In fact, brown rice contains "antinutrients," compounds that bind to the vitamins and minerals, which make some of these nutrients unusable. It is also a myth that sweet potatoes are healthier than white potatoes. Both types contain a variety of nutrients and are a healthy addition to the diet.

Myth: Sweet potatoes are healthier than white potatoes.

Fact: Potatoes can help an individual feel full for a longer period of time, and they contain antioxidants (substances that help control oxidative damage in the body) such as carotenoids (vitamin A precursors), ascorbic acid (vitamin C), and tocopherols (vitamin E). Both are high in B vitamins and phytonutrients (nutrients found in plants) such as polyphenols, alpha-lipoic acid, selenium, lycopene, and many more. Fiber is found on the outside (skin) and inside of both types of potatoes. Sweet potatoes have slightly more fiber per serving, more vitamin A (good for your eyes), manganese (good for wound healing and metabolism), and calcium (good for your bones), but white potatoes have more protein (to build muscles), potassium (for regulating cellular fluid), magnesium (involved in hundreds of bodily systems), and a small amount of iron (for carrying oxygen throughout the body) per serving. Both potatoes offer plenty of nutrient density, and both are recommended for inclusion in the diet.

Myth: Brown rice is healthier than white rice.

Fact: While brown rice has more nutrients, such as magnesium, phosphorus, potassium, manganese, selenium, and copper, it also contains phytates, which act as antinutrients, reducing the body's ability to utilize and absorb the micronutrients it contains. From a health standpoint, this one is genuinely a tie. Neither white rice nor brown rice is superior. Those who consume both white and brown rice get the most nutrients while also remaining flexible.

Our patients often ask, "Why should I force myself to have sugary foods like sweetened cereal or dessert? I can live without that stuff just fine."

Our answer is that to be fully free, you have to understand and trust that your body can eat, digest, and metabolize any and all foods. Modeling this to yourself for each and every food proves this repeatedly. I can have sweetened cereal and nothing bad will happen. I can have a Starbucks Frappuccino and nothing bad will happen. I can have candy and nothing bad will happen. Plus, if you avoid sugar entirely, you are more likely to crave it. Sugar cravings vary by person but tend to escalate when one's overall nutrition is insufficient, when total carbohydrates are low, and when sugar is eliminated from one's diet. This can lead to binge eating. Eventually, you will learn to hear and trust what your body is calling for and respond to its needs accordingly.

Food is so much more than just nutrients. Food is joy, socialization, culture, celebration, family togetherness, holidays, and more. If you only ever ate "whole grains," how would you dine out in restaurants? Or at a friend's house? Or join relatives for homemade latkes? Or enjoy Thanksgiving dinner? The ability to be flexible and eat in a variety of settings is key to being spontaneous and adaptable! The more you can eat different foods in different places, the more you can trust your body and recognize that it can handle anything. Part of rebuilding your relationship with food is finding your true joy and happiness with food again.

It will take expanding your choices to find that joy. Saying yes when you want to say no. Experiencing new food environments. Eating someone else's cooking and seeing that "it's okay" and nothing terrible happened. This is all part of exposure work. But first, we have to find out where the ED is hiding, so we continue to play detective.

For example, many have a list of "safe" foods.These foods might be ones that feel "good" or "healthy." They may be consumed in a repetitive way, daily, without deviation. Safe foods vary by person, and they usually cause very little escalation of anxiety. And the consumption of these safe foods might also be keeping your ED alive.

Safe foods can be those a person trusts and relies on or that someone can tolerate safely without side effects. Some of our neurodivergent patients rely on safe foods as cornerstones in their day. We also have patients that need safe foods that are allergen-free or safe for their gastrointestinal tract. For the sake of this discussion, we are highlighting the repeated decision to choose foods that are perceived as "healthier" than others. This practice perpetuates the ED.

Examples of safe foods may be a protein bar, rice cake, or morning smoothie. Safe snacks might be a granola bar and pear; a safe meal might be grilled chicken breast, brown rice, and steamed broccoli. If you always choose the same safe foods, the ED can stay alive and hide. It's important to expand beyond safe foods to see that all foods can fit and nothing terrible happens when you venture outside your comfort zone.

Though it might feel unnecessary to fight seemingly minor food restrictions, remember that this fight is really about completely obliterating the ED, remnants of which might be lurking in those subtle restrictions. Which foods come to mind that might be holding you back? Can you expand your diet beyond your safe foods?

Are You Eating with Enough Variety?

Even as you progress, it's important to keep assessing your variety. Take a look back at the seven-day food record that you completed in chapter 3. How often are you eating the same breakfast? The same lunch? For example, having a yogurt and an apple might be enough volume for a snack, but if you are having the same snack every day or almost every day, it will likely keep you fearful of snack foods like chips and guacamole or cheese and crackers. Similarly, if you are eating oatmeal every morning for breakfast, is it preventing you from trying a bagel, an egg sandwich, or a seitan and avocado wrap?

Eating a variety of foods helps to ensure flexibility and enables your body get different nutrients from different foods. For example, chicken is low in iron. If you ate only chicken every day, you would be missing out on iron found in red meat. Similarly, if you ate an orange every day, you would get plenty of vitamin C but would miss out on the potassium found in bananas.

A fun and rewarding way to expand what you eat and how you prepare it is to find new recipes. The internet is your friend here! In some cases, using a meal service like Blue Apron, Hello Fresh, Gobble, Freshly, or Home Chef can help push you out of your comfort zone.

SUMMARY OF DETECTIVE WORK

Return to Baseline

What are some old favorites you used to love?

Meals?

Snacks?

Favorite restaurants?

And/or: What would you want to borrow from how you used to eat?

Eating in Community

Can you eat in front of people?

Inner circle?

Extended circle?

Participate in what is being served?

Can you let go of dietary restrictions?

Can you let go of vegetarianism/veganism?

Is there still an overfocus on safe, "clean" foods?

What are your safe foods?

Is there enough variety in what you eat?

Can you increase the variety of foods you eat?

CHAPTER 16

Four Steps to
Freeing Yourself from
Food Fears

FIGHTING FOOD FEARS is hard work, but peace awaits you on the other side. Throughout this chapter, we will take you through four steps for reducing food fears. The first and second step will ask you to systematically understand and uncover what your food fears are. Steps three and four will help you challenge these fears through a process called exposure. Exposing yourself to foods that escalate your anxiety and challenging your food rules lead to a desensitization to the feared item. By chipping away at your food fears, you'll eventually make them disappear. Which brings us to an important point about this process: You get to decide whether and how you work on food exposures. And if you decide to move forward, you get to decide the path.

Step 1: Which Foods Escalate Your Anxiety?

To really know which foods escalate your anxiety, you will need to develop a clear road map of your vulnerabilities. Let's work on creating a list of all those foods. Can you include the findings from your detective work from the previous chapter? Think about food categories like proteins, carbohydrates, fruits, vegetables, fats, snacks, and desserts.

Be as specific as possible. For example, if you write "desserts," can you specify which desserts? Or if you list "red meat," assign rankings for steak, ground beef, meatballs, a burger from a fast-food chain, and a homemade burger, all of which might feel different. Does melted cheese feel different to you than cold cheese? If so, list these items separately! Noting this information will serve to guide you through your exposure work.

Once you have your list, assign a value next to each food to indicate the least to most anxiety-provoking food (0 = not scary at all, 10 = frightening!). This will be your food hierarchy list, which will delineate foods you are least and most scared of. We will come back to this list in "Step 3: Practice a Few Exposures and Challenges Each Week" (page 231). We can start with whichever food feels the easiest. It's fun to add the date next to the ranking so you can track the changes as months go by. If you have been practicing, the anxiety rankings will inevitably decrease. It is extremely exciting to see a marked reduction in anxiety rankings for certain foods or, better yet, crossing foods off your list entirely!

FOOD	RANKING (0–10: 0 LOW ANXIETY, 10 HIGH ANXIETY)

Here is an example of our client Dennis's food hierarchy rankings.

FOOD	RANKING (0–10: 0 LOW ANXIETY, 10 HIGH ANXIETY)
Brownie	1/3/23 → **4**
Bagel	1/3/23 → **6**
Burger	1/3/23 → **6**
Burger and fries from In-N-Out, used to go with friends	1/3/23 → **9**
Fries	1/3/23 → **4**
Chipotle—always used to go with friends	1/3/23 → **5**
Juice	1/3/23 → **4**
Muffin	1/3/23 → **5**
Mayo	1/3/23 → **4**
Pasta	1/3/23 → **7**
Cookie	1/3/23 → **6**
Sugared cereal—grew up eating	1/3/23 → **3**
Chips	1/3/23 → **8**
Crackers	1/3/23 → **5**
Flavored yogurt	1/3/23 → **3**
My mother's baked ziti	1/3/23 → **7**
Snacks: chips, baked goods, desserts, ice cream, bagged snacks	1/3/23 → **8**

Step 2: Which Food Rules Are You Still Following

Food rules are often rooted in diet culture and typically followed without a clear explanation. These rules are often self-imposed and concern what/when you can or cannot eat, how much, and which foods are "allowed" according to your ED. The goal is to enumerate these and then, one by one, *break every single rule!*

Fight back against food rules

- "I must read all the food labels." Can you move beyond foods with nutrition labels? Numbers, tracking, and calorie counting increase obsessiveness and distress around food. Let go of counting. Start small, maybe with a snack.

Fight-back strategy: Buy something at the bakery.

- "I will only eat packaged foods with nutrition labels that tell me the exact calorie amounts." Nutrition labels make it difficult to encounter real-world situations, including travel, restaurants, dinner at a friend's, and dining halls. Labels and pre-portioned foods keep the ED comfortable. Make the ED more uncomfortable.

Fight-back strategy: Go to a restaurant! Or go out for ice cream.

- "I will not eat after 7:00 AM." This implies that something will happen if you eat beyond a certain time. There is no scientific evidence that supports eating at one time versus another. This is driven by diet culture. Placing a time limit on eating interrupts socialization, dating, and traveling, and may even lead to nighttime bingeing. It keeps the ED alive by keeping you from following your meal plan.

Fight-back strategy: Begin to have a snack one hour after that time, and keep pushing it back later and later!

- "I have to measure all my food." Many are dependent on measuring cups and spoons. We want you to go out to eat without measuring!

Fight-back strategy: With the Plate-by-Plate Approach®, no measurements are needed. If you are unable to transition right away to a no-numbers approach, consider measuring one last time—then stop. Assess the portion, and commit to ditching the measuring cups altogether.

- "I will only eat homemade food with my own ingredients." Homemade food keeps you at home.

Fight-back strategy: Go to a friend's house. Then pick a restaurant. Slowly venture out.

What are your food rules?

Examples

I can't eat past 7:00 PM.

I can't eat out twice in one day.

I can't have dessert in the afternoon.

I can't have dessert if I don't work out.

I can't drink juice, only water.

I can only have homemade desserts.

I can't have packaged snacks.

Steps 3 & 4: Exposure, Exposure, Exposure!

Working on eradicating food fears takes courage and persistence. It takes a firm belief that this process will work and in the effort to fight against a resistant and unrelenting ED. If you are interested in putting energy toward rebuilding your relationship with food, the journey will involve a technique psychologists call "exposure." This means facing and experiencing your fears. This process is hard and may increase your anxiety in the short term. There may be tears, failed attempts, and feelings of wanting to give up, but what waits for you on the other side is complete food freedom.

Exposure therapy is typically used to treat anxiety disorders, including panic disorder, certain phobias, and obsessive-compulsive disorder. Exposure works by confronting something that creates an escalation of anxiety and allowing a person, through repeated exposures to that trigger, to acclimate or "habituate" to it. This means that the more someone is exposed to something scary, the less fear they experience in its presence over time.

For example, one of our patients reported feeling terrified to be alone at night in her apartment. She was one of four siblings, used to always being around people. As a young adult, she had three roommates and found it oddly quiet when they were all busy and out at the same time. She would stay out all night, bouncing between various friends' houses until she knew one of her roommates had returned home. Sometimes this went on at all hours of the night. She hated it but was too scared to be home alone, until one day, when she felt weak and feverish, she had to lie down. She needed to go home, but all her roommates were gone! She was too sick to care and went into the apartment alone. She did it. When she felt better, she thought "That wasn't so bad." Being alone, even when sick, showed her that her fears were far worse than the reality.

The fear of certain foods, the worry or preoccupation about how food is prepared, or despair that food is unhealthy is a form of anxiety. Repeated exposures to any of these circumstances or to a feared food allow you to become desensitized to these fears over time. This allows you to eventually become comfortable, even if initially reluctant or avoidant. By confronting food fears and becoming more comfortable with these experiences, you are eventually able to build experiences that reduce fear. The repeated aspect of the exposure is a learning process; instead of the food being attached to the belief that something bad will happen, the food becomes associated with the experience that all will be okay.

Continuing to avoid these foods reinforces the negative thoughts and feelings they elicit. Avoidance prevents you from getting the chance to experience (and thus learn) that you can tolerate the food. The more you avoid ordering ice cream from an ice cream shop or a burrito from Chipotle, the scarier it remains in your mind. It's only when you challenge it that you can see, "Wow, that wasn't so scary!"

To be clear, most people are not initially excited about this part of recovery. Many will admit, "I actually *wanted* to have the cookies I had been baking for others," but most will also say they were terrified to eat them. "Sometimes so many exposures feel overwhelming. I would need to take a break for a few weeks. Did I look different? Did my clothes feel different? It was like I became paranoid," one client described.

"Feeling terrified" tends not to be something that most want to sign up for. But unless you challenge the belief that eating a bagel will immediately make you gain five pounds, the thought will intensify in your mind. (This exposure can be twofold: eat the bagel and see nothing terrible happen or gain weight and realize the feelings associated with weight gain are tolerable.) Challenging misguided thoughts drains their power.

We should warn you that we have seen people *lose weight* during times of food exposures. This is never the intention, but it can happen for several reasons. For one, many overemphasize the impact of their exposure. A snack like ice cream—which might feel really challenging for some—can cause people to restrict themselves at other times of the day. Many compensate for a food exposure at a meal by eliminating the next snack. "This *must* count for extra" when really it wouldn't. We have had people consider food exposure at snack as "double" the normal snack amount. But a challenge snack isn't double your regular snack! Ice cream wouldn't necessarily count for more than your "safe" snack of yogurt and granola or an apple and peanut butter.

Case Study: Cooper

Cooper was heading out on a weeklong retreat. He had been struggling to expand variety and was eating the same safe foods each day. Eating in this new environment would be tough. He decided to go but knew it would be hard. When he returned, he was gushing about all his new food experiences: chocolate, breads, pasta with sauce on it, new meats! It was an amazing learning experience. Yet when he saw his medical doctor, his weight had dropped precipitously and his heart rate was dangerously low. What happened? Most likely, while he had tried many new foods, he wasn't eating *enough* of these foods. This was nonetheless a great launchpad from which to move forward.

Why are exposures worth it? Several readers wrote to share the following.

- "Now I get excited about the food I'm going to eat instead of dreading it."
- "Socializing with friends is so much more enjoyable."
- "I get to enjoy flavors I haven't tasted in so long!"
- "I no longer feel envy/anger toward other people I see eating the foods I truly want to eat."
- "It helps me clear out more brain space to experience more interesting things."

- "Now I enjoy flipping through a restaurant menu and having a ton of choices."

- "When I started running again, I needed flexible food options, more carbs, and lower-volume foods. I couldn't have done that with my existing food fears and I'm grateful to explore a new sport."

- "It's given me moments and memories with my husband that I otherwise would have missed."

- "Even though some days are harder than others, my view of myself is so much more positive now."

Step 3: Practice a Few Exposures and Challenges Each Week

Now the fun begins. Looking at your excellent detective work, let's get started. You can arrange your food-fear rankings from least scary to most scary, creating a hierarchy. Then you can decide which foods to start with. Generally, individuals start with the least scary foods. But there is no official rule of thumb that says you have to start with the least scary; some have chosen to get the most scary foods over with first, and studies support that it's safe to start with the foods that are most anxiety provoking. It's like ripping off a Band-Aid. Most people choose to start with the relatively easy foods first and "prove" they can be successful, then build on that.

In the example provided for Dennis on page 226, the following least-scary items are listed.

WEEK 1

Flavored yogurt	3
Sugared cereal	3
Mayonnaise	4
Fries	4
Brownie	4

Challenge food rule: I won't eat past 7:00 PM.

The number of foods tried, and the frequency of exposures conducted, depend on how many exposures you think you can handle and how motivated you are. You are fully in the driver's seat here. You can decide how fast this moves, if at all. The more you practice, the faster your journey to food freedom. It will be a balancing act to conduct exposures without getting too overwhelmed, since we know exposures can increase anxiety. Each exposure will require repeat experiences, while shifting the circumstances slightly, to build comfort and habituation.

Step 4: Repeat Exposures to the Food, in Several Different Circumstances

At the heart of it, successful exposure work requires repetition. As you practice repetition, can you shift the circumstances? If you tried a homemade burger, can you try a burger from a restaurant next time? If you are trying brownies, you might think about how many different ways you can eat one. You might first try baking brownies at home, then buy one from a bakery, and then from a coffee shop. Repeated attempts are important in knocking down the fear and creating new positive experiences. When you experience the challenge and see that "nothing bad happened," you are collecting evidence that can be used to challenge the original irrational thought. Research studying limited eaters shows it can take fifteen to twenty exposures before someone can convert a food from a dislike to a like.[1] Each exposure is meant to be done many times, in many forms, and fully experienced (swallowed).

You can use a form like the Food Exposure Checklist to track which and how many exposures were done. You can find a link to download this form in the resources section on page 303.

FOOD EXPOSURE CHECKLIST

TRIED?	FOOD	NUMBER OF TRIES							COMMENTS

In the earlier example, Dennis decided to work a variety of flavored yogurts into his meal plan. He planned to consume different flavored yogurts on different days. The repetition is key, as is planning to do the exposure in several different ways. For example, he might include peach flavored yogurt in a smoothie, and a different brand of strawberry yogurt as part of a snack on a different day. Typically, it will take multiple experiences before the anxiety level will be reduced. He might also simultaneously be working on reducing anxiety around sugared cereal.

Case Study: Naya

Naya was working hard on food exposures with her dietitian. Here is a snapshot of how her anxiety decreased over time: 11/1/2020 (Day 1), 2/25/21 (3 months later), and 5/17/21 (3 months later).

Foods that Escalate Naya's Anxiety (10 = high anxiety, 1 = low anxiety)			
Naan	11/1/2020 → 3	2/25/21 → 3	5/17/21 → 0
White rice	11/1/2020 → 5	2/25/21 → 1	5/17/21 → 0
Brown rice	11/1/2020 → 2	2/25/21 → 1	5/17/21 → 0
Daal with oil	11/1/2020 → 5	2/25/21 → 2	5/17/21 → 0
Pasta with sauce	11/1/2020 → 6	2/25/21 → 2-3	5/17/21 → 0
Juices/lassi	11/1/2020 → 7	2/25/21 → 4-5	5/17/21 → 1
Pastry	11/1/2020 → 7-8	2/25/21 → 2-3	5/17/21 → 1
Brownie	11/1/2020 → 7	2/25/21 → 2	5/17/21 → 1
Filled donut	11/1/2020 → 8-9	2/25/21 → 3-4	5/17/21 → 0.5
Ice cream from home (measuring)	11/1/2020 → 6	2/25/21 → 6	5/17/21 → 0
Ice cream out	11/1/2020 → 7	2/25/21 → 2	5/17/21 → 0
Chips	11/1/2020 → 7	2/25/21 → 3	5/17/21 → 0
Prepackaged foods (e.g., stuffing)	11/1/2020 → 8	2/25/21 → 2-3	5/17/21 → 1

After Naya had worked on her food fears and anxieties for 6 months, they were significantly lower.

    0 out of 10 for 8 foods

    1 out of 10 for 4 foods

    0.5 out of 10 for 1 food

This was amazing though not surprising because she had practiced exposures over and over.

By this point, she felt empowered and confident around food.

Family Food Experiments

Family food experiments are a fun way to work on exposures in a group setting, for those with limited food preferences such as ARFID. Pick something like chocolate to start, or apples, or grapes. Find four or five varieties of the food you have chosen. Examine each variety one at a time, and assess as a group the color of the food and how it looks, tastes, feels, and smells. Which is your favorite? With social support, this allows for non-pressured food exploration. If this goes well, you can expand to another food.

What Makes an Exposure More Successful?

Here are a few factors that will maximize the likelihood that your exposure will be successful.

1. **Environment:** Where are you doing the exposure? Are you in a calm setting, at the kitchen table, using a plate, fork, and knife? Or are you in the car, eating out of containers, or on your lap? It can be stressful to not be able to plate the food or to feel rushed.

2. **Timing:** Have you given yourself enough time? Eating as part of exposures might take longer to muster up the courage or deal with your feelings afterward. If you are rushing around, this might make the morning/afternoon/evening even more difficult.

3. **Clothing:** Many have reported feeling triggered by what they were wearing the day of an exposure. For example, Sasha was wearing a tight skirt and a fitted top on the afternoon she was set to try an exposure. She knew if she had changed into more casual clothing, trying a feared food would have been easier. She was self-conscious about how her body felt in her outfit as she was doing the exposure, and she couldn't move past it. Of course, this is something to revisit, but it was too much to experience the food exposure and the body image distress at the same time.

It's Not Working

If any of this feels prohibitively anxiety-provoking or isn't working for you, we suggest bringing the exposures to a session with your therapist. Many people have significant feeding difficulties, troubles with food textures, smells, and temperature, and simply trying foods on their own won't work. They will likely need more one-on-one intensive-feeding therapy. Some people will need physical therapy, occupational therapy, and other services to reach their goals.

CHAPTER 17

———◁———

Navigating Real Life

NAVIGATING LIFE OUTSIDE your ED requires continued exposures in a variety of settings. This helps bolster your confidence around a variety of foods and situations, so you say "Yes!" without fear. In chapters 15 and 16, you worked hard on identifying and tackling your food fears. Exposure allowed you to reduce individual food fears and break some long-standing food rules. Now, we will help you explore the other challenges that arise as you engage more with life. These challenges include going to restaurants, traveling, managing times of sickness, returning to work, dealing with the effects of surgery, and navigating the holidays. As you challenge the ED, you will continue to reduce food anxiety and build flexibility. To be successful at this stage, it will be important to stay on track with the Plate-by-Plate Approach®, despite obstacles and transitions.

Here are some criteria we consider to assess who might experience success with meal outings. This is not to say that if you don't meet these criteria you can't go out to eat, but it will certainly make it easier.

- Nearing or in goal weight range, or weight stable for those who don't need to gain weight
- Medically stable
- Normalized hormones (estrogen, testosterone); e.g., having regular menstrual cycles (for those not experiencing perimenopause or menopause)
- Compliant with meal plans

- Flexible with food
- Up for the adventure
- Committed, even if slightly, to recovery

Consideration for Meal Explorations

As you begin to consider exploring meals in new places, it's always good to check in with yourself about your level of readiness, and how *you* feel about it. Troubleshooting any potential feelings around the new experience and potential barriers to being successful is important to help you succeed. For example, if a client shared, "I am nervous about getting distracted at the concert and not being able to eat my snack," we might suggest having the snack before or after, rather than during the concert. These are great topics to talk through with your treatment team.

Here are some questions to consider before embarking on any new food experience.

- Has your ED receded enough to allow you to be successful at the meal?
- Have you had success at home when you've been without support?
- Do you think you will succeed with this eating experience?
- Do you feel ready for this challenge?
- Do you know the meal plan well enough to easily plate an appropriate meal?
- Does this challenge come at a good time for you? If begun during a stressful time like a family move or a difficult work period, food explorations are less likely to be successful.

Restaurants

Often those with EDs feel an escalation in anxiety when eating out in restaurants. Confronting your fears can help reduce or eliminate them! Restaurant exposure requires flexibility. If you've practiced eating one kind of dish at home—for example, spaghetti and meatballs—and found the meal to be a successful, then you might be ready to try this dish at your local Italian restaurant. By first trying challenging meals at home, you are practicing the skills necessary to be successful away from home.

Early in one's recovery, navigating restaurants can be daunting, especially if you have not done enough of the exposure work discussed in chapters 15 and 16. The ED might be fighting against what looks and sounds good versus what the "healthier" option is. Choosing from among many menu offerings can be overwhelming. If possible, de-escalate the anxiety in the moment by calmly looking at the menu ahead of time. What sounds good *to you*? What did you order at this restaurant pre-ED? Chicken alfredo and a side salad? Go for it!

The ED might also be so thrilled to be going out to dinner that you might wish to order more than usual. Keeping up with food exposures will help to make food just food, so that all food is allowed and part of your life. Eating regularly throughout the day will help manage your hunger and satiety levels. Do not try to "save your appetite" for the restaurant meal (that's a diet culture trap). This will backfire and cause you to walk into the meal feeling ravenous, making you more likely to binge or bypass your body's natural stopping place.

Unless you have food allergies and intolerances, consider accepting the food as it has been prepared. The ED can be very demanding: "I'll have the turkey club sandwich, on sliced wheat bread, no aioli, no bacon, no cheese, no avocado. And can you please replace the fries with a side salad and hold the dressing?" Being able to accept food as it arrives— and seeing that nothing bad happens as a result of experiencing the unknown—allows you to become a fearless and confident eater. This exposure to restaurant meals is important; you will feel less anxiety at restaurants if you can practice this over time. These are helpful skills to harness when traveling, going away to college, or going, well, anywhere.

A word of caution about going to a restaurant and "barely eating." Having a nutritionally inadequate meal at a restaurant, perhaps only a salad or an appetizer, could set your recovery back. Even if you're out of the medical danger zone, you are still recovering. We don't want to allow the ED in, even for one meal. This could affect the way your mind thinks about your next meal, and the one thereafter. Maybe for you it won't have a huge effect, or maybe it will. We don't want to give the ED an opportunity to thrive.

As you navigate different types of restaurant meals, ask yourself, are all food groups present and is it enough? The priority when eating out is to make sure the plate is adequate, and when restaurants don't have certain food items, it is important to add extras (from whatever food group you want) to cover for the volume expected on that plate. For example, when going to Japanese or Chinese restaurants, there is usually not an obvious dairy source to add to the plate. In that case, you can add a different drink instead (juice or soda) or add an extra item onto your plate, such as an egg roll or edamame.

Restaurant Planning Worksheet

	GRAINS/ STARCHES	PROTEIN	FRUIT/ VEGGIES	FATS	DAIRY/DAIRY ALTERNATIVE (or other food group to cover)
Chinese					
Japanese					
Thai					
Burgers					
Deli					
Italian					
Indian					
Korean					
Mexican					
German					
Greek					

As you work through different types of eating establishments, don't forget about the key aspects of exposure: repetition and changing the circumstances. Plan to visit all your old favorites and to include a diversity of cuisines, such as Mexican, Japanese, Chinese, Thai, Indian, Italian, and whatever else is nearby! We see this as a "food exposure intensive." Seeking a wide range of experiences is the goal. And while it obviously costs money to eat in different restaurants, this same goal can be accomplished by the cooking of different friends and relatives. Or do a food swap: You cook, they cook. Or look for different street fairs, food trucks, or festivals where you can get more reasonably priced food. It's an investment in your future food freedom. Check the box if you've eaten in the following types of restaurants and keep track of how many times you've been there.

FOOD EXPOSURE CHECKLIST

TRIED?	FOOD	NUMBER OF TRIES								COMMENTS
	Chinese restaurant 1									
	Chinese restaurant 2									
	Japanese restaurant 1									
	Japanese restaurant 2									
	Mexican food 1									
	Mexican food 2									
	Pizza place 1									
	Pizza place 2									
	Burger from restaurant									
	Burger from home									
	Snadwich shop 1									
	Sandwich shop 2									
	Buffet line 1									
	Bugget line 2									

Pizza!

For many of our patients, eating pizza is an important part of socialization, whether it be at parties, meetings, or other events. It's one of those foods that you'll be around more than you may realize. Pizza might feel scary, but it doesn't have to be! Learning how much pizza makes a sufficient meal and practicing eating it over and over again will help you gain the confidence to master it.

Become a pizza connoisseur by going to different pizza restaurants. Thin-crust pizza is different from deep-dish pizza, and one pizzeria is different from the next. We recommend starting where it feels comfortable. Pictured here are two small slices of pizza, which equals one slice of New York–style pizza. A typical meal might include 2 slices of NY pizza (4 small slices of this pizza pictured here). But start where it feels right for you, and don't be surprised if you still want more!

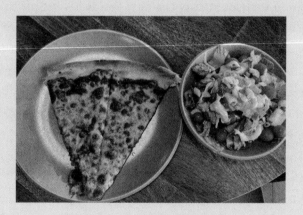

Going Back to Work

Reintegrating yourself into the work setting, or simply trying to keep up, can be taxing. There might be work meals, drinks, birthdays, and talk about weight loss and dieting. This can be triggering and stressful. What can you do? Let's break it down.

Work meals are a good time to practice exposure. The more you have been practicing, the easier this will be for you. Can you look at the menu ahead of time and choose an entrée that sounds good? Social meals with people with whom you might not feel so comfortable are already stressful, so it might make sense to choose an entrée that you feel like you can master rather than something that feels challenging.

We have had many patients bring their own meals to conferences or work dinners. For some, there may be a medical need like a food allergy. For others, it may be a practice of safety. Conferences can be loud and overwhelming. Some of our neurodiverse patients become overstimulated in these settings and rely on foods that are comforting. However, if you don't fall into this category, you might want to explore whether or how to participate in the work event. This will require practicing your exposures first.

You might bill work meals to the company/business, and if you are at risk of bingeing, this can add another tricky dimension. Being able to charge a meal to the company credit card may cause you to "save up" their calories for this meal. We strongly encourage you to avoid the temptation to restrict during the day; this leads people to bypass their body's natural stopping place when it comes to listening to their satiety cues. Stay on track with your regular meals and snacks, otherwise these free work outings can end up being a stressful experience all-around and a trigger for anyone struggling to manage their ED behaviors.

If your colleagues are discussing their diets around you, don't hesitate to ask them to take their diet talk elsewhere. Keto talk or intermittent fasting talk is not only annoying; it's triggering, especially while you are working hard to stick to your plan of regular meals and snacks. The ED wants very badly to latch on to dieting, and on a down day, it can be hard to fight it. But when you are feeling strong, tell them, "We don't all want to hear about how many calories you ate today." Feel free to be as honest as you want. The more honest you are, the more people tend to understand. Shut down diet culture, otherwise, it will keep poking at you day in and day out.

Travel

Whether it's for vacation, business, sports, or to visit family members, traveling is an inevitable part of life. Travel brings challenges, such as limited food options on a long car or plane ride, new foods, the need to be spontaneous with food, different time zones, and an altered meal schedule. It often comes with an unpredictable schedule and an uncertainty around the food (what it is, where it comes from, how it is prepared)—all of which can be hard for someone actively struggling with an ED. There is also additional food required to cover the increased energy expenditure from sightseeing and walking around all day. These adjustments can prove difficult.

Travel is exciting, and most feel it's worth it. The further along you are in your ED recovery, the easier it is, as your palate has presumably been expanded and your medical stability will have increased. This is important, because if a trip does not go well, you might end up in a medically fragile situation. We've had clients who traveled internationally and fainted or had to return home urgently mid-trip, with doctors first having to assess whether the person was sufficiently medically stable to fly home. We've had families who needed to check in with hotel doctors, who often aren't trained in ED management, or who needed to seek out hospitals while in remote locations. We've had clients get admitted to a hospital immediately upon returning home, and we've seen countless trips ruined (and money wasted) because the individual wasn't ready to navigate the food and felt miserable.

If you travel in the early stages of ED treatment, it may be safer to start with a shorter trip that is not far from home. Here are some things to consider.

1. If you can't add more food than you are currently consuming, don't travel. You will need more food and more hydration for your days of sightseeing or working.

2. Bring familiar snacks with you. You don't know what snacks will be available at your destination. Bring some portable, non-refrigerated options.

3. In your checked luggage, bring Ensure Plus or BOOST Plus (1 or 2 minimum for each day you'll be away) just in case.

4. Don't underestimate the effect of hanging around the pool or ocean all day. Vacations can be active! One of our clients was an athlete who was surprised to see she had lost weight after a trip. She didn't account

for the long walks to dinner (round-trip) each night and much of the walking she did while sightseeing. It all adds up and needs to be accounted for.

5.   Consider adding drinks like juice, milk, or smoothies to boost your meal plan. This is easy to do, universally available, and doesn't contribute to a lot of fullness.

Holiday Meals

It's common for an ED to prevent someone from eating their favorite holiday foods. Whether it's noodle kugel or pumpkin pie, an individual who is still actively struggling with an ED might feel anxious in the presence of these foods. When foods surface once a year, exposure can be hard to practice. But fear not! Confidence comes from exposure to other foods throughout the year. You learn through other exposures that your body can handle new foods, unknown foods, foods with sugar, foods with fats, and everything in between. When you're fighting for recovery, repeated exposures are necessary to reduce anxiety and increase comfort around different types of foods. It's a very exciting milestone to join a holiday meal and participate fully.

Holiday meals may be overwhelming. There may be a lot of people present whom you haven't seen for a while. You might be pressured to answer a lot of questions: "How are you doing?" "How are you feeling?" "You look better." This line of conversation can be triggering and overwhelming. Be sure to troubleshoot some of these topics in advance. What do you want to share? If people say you "look good," how will your recovery voice take that? If it feels too overwhelming, have a safe exit plan. Where can you go to escape?

Most likely, holiday meals offer a variety of delicious foods. For tips on how to navigate plating a festive meal, see the box that follows.

We use this strategy to follow the Plate-by-Plate Approach® at buffets, dining halls, parties, holiday meals, and many other circumstances.

· First, scan the food. What do you see? What are you drawn to? What feels and sounds good?

· Then decide what protein you want to start with and add it to your plate.

· Next, choose a starch that sounds good and fill it up according to whichever plate you are using (50% or 33% starch plate).

· Add a vegetable.

· Is there a source of dairy you can add?

· If not, find another food group that you can add to cover for volume; this can be an appetizer or dessert.

· Don't forget to fill the plate up completely!

Religious Dietary Changes and Fasting

There may also be religious events that involve altering the diet. Those who are Catholic may fast on Ash Wednesday and Good Friday and abstain from meat on Fridays during Lent. Muslims who follow Ramadan will fast from dawn to sunset for a month. Fasting is common on the Jewish holiday Yom Kippur and on other holy days. Additional religions and philosophies that practice fasting include Buddhism, Protestantism, Islam, Taoism, Jainism, and Hinduism. Fasting can last for just a few hours or even a few weeks.

Despite these deeply meaningful practices, it is often not medically or psychologically recommended for those with EDs. The decision to abstain from a religious fast is not taken lightly. Fasting is meant for those of "able body and mind." A careful evaluation by one's treatment team is recommended.

Fasting can be appealing to the ED, and it can make it hard for you to return to normal eating. Some may fail to catch up on the nutrition they missed when fasting, and thus lose ground. It's often not worth risking until the ED is fully in your rearview mirror. Here are some questions to consider when evaluating if it's safe for you to fast.

- Are you medically stable?

- Is your recovery solid? (Would an alteration in your diet derail your recovery?)

- Are you able to increase meals before and after fasting to make up for missed nutrition without too much stress?

When You're Not Ready for a Must-Attend Event

We have heard about thousands of these events through our patients' stories—whether it's the annual dance performance, a backpacking excursion you've been planning for months, or a once-in-a-lifetime meet and greet with an admired celebrity in another city. What to do? If you are not medically stable and/or unable to eat at your destination, then we urge you to consider skipping the event. If you are set to weather the uncertainty that travel brings, you may be setting yourself up for failure. Attending an event, even one that involves only a meal or two, can cause you to backtrack and allow the ED to come roaring back. Despite the can't-miss event, we ask you to discount the emotions around the event and make a decision that's best for your recovery.

If you must attend but don't think you are ready, you should consider a strategy to optimize how you will manage the food. For example, perhaps you plan to have supported meals before and after the event. Perhaps you can plan to eat with someone at the event. Though it is not ideal to attend an event prematurely, if the event is important enough, it will be imperative that you complete meals prior to the event and during the event. Making a game plan will help keep you on track with your nutrition, while minimizing the risks associated with navigating difficult food experiences.

Sickness

Sickness can be very disruptive for those with an ED. Whether it's the flu, COVID-19, or a stomach virus, being out of your routine, feeling slower or weaker than usual, perhaps spending time on bedrest and off your eating schedule, can awaken the ED. It might start with a suppressed appetite, and your weight might decrease a little. That might be all that's needed to start the cycle of the ED mindset. This can come as a surprise to those who had been cruising along and feeling like they were in a solid place in recovery. *How did I get here?* one of our clients asks of her recent experience with multiple bouts of illness.

Recovery from both the illness and the ED resurgence requires careful attention to fueling. It requires eating even when you don't feel you need or want to. It might mean that the plate doesn't have all food groups present, or that you consume more fluids such as soups, juice, Popsicles, and smoothies, and that's okay. Experiment with foods and fluids you *can* eat while sick, and once you're better, get back on track as soon as possible.

Sickness can suppress hunger cues and may create the need for a mini period of nutritional rehabilitation. This means that you might need to regain weight, restore vital signs, and repair metabolism—but for a shorter period this time. Don't despair; you did it once, and you can do it again. You know what the journey back looks like!

The expectation is that, while it may be uncomfortable, you *can* complete meals and snacks, and prolonging this step is likely to compromise your recovery. It is also important that you notify your treatment team if you are sick. Your medical provider may want to see you to check your weight and vital signs, to be sure you are not becoming medically unstable due to illness. Resilience is key here. We are not immune to getting sick. What counts is how we respond. This is a chance to build resilience in the face of your ED. Fight back by getting your favorite foods together, rallying support, calling your therapist, scheduling appointments with your treatment team, and setting lunch dates for accountability. Responding in these ways says, "I will not let this eating disorder come back into my life!"

Here are some things to consider when you are sick.

1. Try your best to eat regularly every few hours (maybe even more frequently than usual). This means you might be eating eight times

a day if you are unable to eat your usual-size meals. That might be hard for the ED, but you need to take care of yourself!

2. Hydrate with water—and, yes, juices, Gatorade, and soups. The ED might not like this, but that's okay. The ED doesn't have your best interest at heart.

3. Calorically dense options will help by maximizing nutrition in every bite.

4. Consider less bulk during this time (fewer fruits and vegetables). Think of the Plate-by-Plate® guidelines (25% of the plate) as a good guide for fruits/vegetables. Juice and smoothies might be a simpler way to get in vitamins and minerals.

5. Keep a close eye on your weight, especially if you have had trouble staying at an appropriate weight for your body.

6. Recruit support. Can someone help with meal prep or food shopping?

Surgery and Dental Woes

Patients in treatment for their ED might require a surgery, such as an ACL repair or knee replacement, or a dental intervention: braces, wisdom tooth surgery, a root canal, a crown, and so on. These procedures can have a big impact on recovery and on one's ability to eat! We have seen such procedures derail recovery for some (irrespective of diagnosis or weight).

Here are some items to consider before signing up for any surgical or dental interventions.

1. Are you medically stable? Surgery is always risky, but do you have stable and consistent enough vitals to withstand whatever the difficulties in eating might present?

2. Can you imagine yourself successfully following the recommended diet post-surgery or post-intervention? In the case of most dental procedures, especially surgery, this usually includes soft foods and liquids like ice cream, smoothies, shakes, and yogurt. If that alone

is too anxiety provoking, then stop right there and proceed no further. You need to be ready to fuel yourself during this time, and not eating or undereating should not be considered a viable option, even if only temporarily. This can be a very slippery slope, which can lead to dangerous consequences.

3. Changing one's diet is incredibly triggering for most people with an ED. Even if items 1 and 2 sound okay, you might want to consider how altering your diet might affect you. The mindset might become, "Well, I ate a little less on Tuesday, so I won't eat as much today . . ." And before you know it, the ED has swept in. This is often surprising and distressing to the patient and their family, who are surprised that the ED resurfaced so quickly.

It may never feel like the "right time" to schedule your surgery. But the best time would be when life is least stressful, not during a major transition, not during peak sports season, not during a big move or a major life event. Aim for when your mood feels most stable, and when you have support around you.

As you prepare to go out into the world, look around and see what areas still need work. What has been missed? As we have explored food fears, food rules, restaurants, travel, sickness, work, and major life events, where are the little places the ED still hides? This might be something that only you know. Find those places and fight back against where the ED might be breathing beneath the surface. For example, are you still measuring your food? Are you only allowing yourself to eat mini bagels or grocery store bagels, which have nutrition labels? Are you only allowing yourself to eat brown rice and never white rice? Have you continued to avoid going to a bakery?

We'll say it again: Find where the ED still exists, and fight back.

CHAPTER 18

Increasing Body Satisfaction

MANY ASK, "What will my body look like in recovery?" The answer, believe it or not, matters *less* as you recover *more*. For example, once your broken leg fully heals, you just stop thinking about it all the time. Other things take over to steer you through your day. The focus shifts to new questions. "What might it be like to redefine my identity beyond things having to do with my body, like who I am and not what I look like?

Nutrition and sleep are foundational pillars of body image work. It's important before doing this work that you are sufficiently nourished and weight-restored. Body image distress stems from cognitions, and to shift those thoughts, the brain has to be in a fully nourished state. Skipping meals, dieting, and energy deficiencies cause negative effects on mood, concentration, and reasoning. Similarly, if you're sleep deprived, it's hard to feel great about anything, especially yourself: mood suffers, energy decreases, and your immune system and body image are compromised. Doesn't everything feel worse when you are tired? Starting from a place of being re-nourished, weight restored, and well rested allows you to approach body image work from a more solid footing; otherwise, as you try to apply skills and tools, the structure will collapse quickly without a strong foundation. When ready, you can start to improve body image by addressing your beliefs ("I will be compassionate with my body, even if I can't accept it yet"), feelings, and behaviors.

How you see your body, relate to your body, and live in your body is unique to you. To "embody" is to give a body a spirit (according to Merriam-Webster). Many people with EDs feel disembodied (or separate from their body, as if it's not their own). Finding a way to relate to your body and inhabit it again can be daunting but also extremely rewarding.

How might you begin to relate to your own body? In her TEDx talk "Lose Hate Not Weight," Virgie Tovar, author, activist, and one of the nation's leading experts on weight-based discrimination and body image, talks about "jiggling" her body as a young child. She describes the elation she experienced as she would move through her house and jiggle the fat on her body in utter appreciation for its magic. "Jiggle like it's 1999," she tells her readers in *The Body Positive Journal*.

We live in a culture in which thin bodies are praised and fat bodies are discriminated against. Advertisements; medical recommendations; and advice from teachers, coaches, and parents are thin-centric. Intergenerational harm from the discrimination toward larger bodies and the effects of diet culture run deep. We are hardwired to fit in. This causes us to shrink ourselves to take up less space. Weight loss and dieting rob you of your essence, mood, and who you really are, diminishing your greatest gifts. All of this unfurls while the $72 billion weight loss industry and $534 billion beauty industry sell you the idea that you aren't good enough.[1] Who could blame you for finding it hard to accept your body?

Through a lifetime of exposure to media, as well as social norms that idealize thin bodies, you have been conditioned to constantly compare your body to others (both *real* bodies and *fake* ones—i.e., Photoshopped). You might be angry that you are no longer "allowed" to diet (because it fuels the ED). You might be grieving your sick and thinner body and the loss of a life you hoped your smaller body might have given you. And you might be experiencing a lot of distress as you fight through your ED and land here—the place your body is supposed to be once the cycle of dieting and ED behaviors have ended. In this chapter, we will focus on providing you with tools you can use to repair your relationship with your body.

Take a Pause

Pausing is helpful for interrupting intrusive rumination, commonly seen with body image distress. On days or moments when you are struggling with your body, stop and ask yourself, What am I feeling? Where am I feeling it? This pause can stop the difficult feelings, the depleting energy, and give you the chance to interrupt the rumination. The pause acts as a form of emotional regulation, stopping the negativity right in its tracks. It also gives you the choice of what to do next.

Negative self-talk, judgment, and self-loathing are like having an abusive relationship with yourself. You certainly wouldn't talk that way to a friend. Begin to interrupt yourself, or cut yourself off, when those words slip easily off your tongue. The goal, of course, is to recognize when this is happening, to lessen the amount of self-inflicted pain. Connie Sobczak, cofounder of The Body Positive, shares, "I want to have a safe place inside of me. If I am mean to myself, then my home isn't safe. I want to have nonviolent communication with myself."

Often this critical voice can be more vocal when we're experiencing other underlying emotions. What is underneath those words for you? Uncovering what's underneath is often the exploration that occurs in therapy or by doing your own explorations in the moment. When you find yourself being particularly critical, you might ask yourself, what do I need right now? What might I be feeling or longing for in those moments?

You might recognize that you are experiencing a sense of heightened fear or anxiety. In those moments you might feel fearful about your future, or insecure about whether you are a good enough mother or partner, or you may feel isolated and alone, and wonder if you will ever be accepted. Once you can recognize the underlying feeling for body image distress, it becomes (somewhat) easier to eliminate the negative emotion toward one's body. This is a practice, and not a finished product.

Gratitude, Body Tolerance, Appreciation

The art of body appreciation is anything but linear. And it's certainly not perfect. Accepting your body's "flaws" or imperfections takes work to stop the barrage of negative body image thoughts and find a different narrative.

Appreciating your body is different from feeling positive about your body. Here, you might simply appreciate what your body can do.

Studies show that gratitude practices increase body appreciation and, notably, block negative, toxic emotions.[2] This is especially helpful on bad body image days, when you can't appreciate your body directly. A gratitude practice is identifying the things in your life for which you are grateful. This practice may have nothing to do with your body specifically; it is a deliberate review of the past, which helps to increase positivity. A general practice of gratitude has been shown to reduce depression and stress and increase joy and pleasure, improve sleep, and aid immune function.[3] As you keep a gratitude journal each day, you might begin to appreciate small things you previously didn't notice—a smile from a passerby, gratitude for catching a ride with someone during a rainstorm, appreciation for the support of your sibling who loves and supports you no matter what.

What might your gratitude practice look like?

When your body image is struggling, it can be helpful to shift your gaze to some of the body's constant, unseen functions. This might sound like the following.

- Thank you, heart, for keeping me alive and allowing me to love.
- Thank you, brain, for allowing me to learn, to think critically, and to remember.
- Thank you, bones, for supporting my body weight, for giving me structure, and storing essential minerals like calcium and phosphorus.
- Thank you, nose, for allowing me to smell the flowers, to take in the scent of my loved ones, to smell the aromas associated with taste in food, and to breathe deeply.
- Thank you, hands, for allowing me to touch, hold, and give.
- Thank you, middle finger, for allowing me to tell off anyone who doesn't appreciate me for me.
- Thank you, mouth, for allowing me to eat, drink, taste, chew, speak, smile, and kiss the ones I love.

- Thank you, legs, for allowing me to move, dance, walk, hike, climb, and swim.
- Thank you, ears, for letting me take in the sweet sounds of nature, listen to music, and hear the words all around me.
- Thank you, eyes, for allowing me to see the world's beauty.
- Thank you, fat, for keeping me alive, providing me with energy, and protecting my organs.

If you cannot align with "appreciating" your body, the concept of "body tolerance" might feel more suitable. That would sound like, "This is *my* body, the only one I have." For a slightly more motivated angle, you could add, "And I will work on accepting it."

Get Rid of Old Clothes and Find Clothing That Works for You Now

The changes you see in your body, while uncomfortable, are necessary; they mean that your body is doing what it needs to. You must trust this process and be patient while your body achieves balance and stability. You may need new clothes, a task you've likely been dreading. Shopping can be a source of great pleasure or a fraught experience, depending on your relationship with your body. For an individual recovering from an ED, it will likely be the latter.

Some patients complain of clothes that "don't fit." Whether they actually don't fit or you don't like the fit, it's probably time to ditch them. Nan Shaw, LCSW, FBT, CEDS-S, says, "Get rid of all clothes with 'memory.' Meaning, clothes that 'used to fit this way, and now you feel they don't,' whether accurate or not."

While shopping might be stressful, remember, finding something that feels good for your body—regardless of the size on the label—is the goal. It's amazing how much a new outfit can add pep to your step. Clothing does not need to be expensive. There are amazing thrift stores in most towns as well as online, where you can find gently used clothing at affordable prices. So, if you don't feel ready to buy a whole new wardrobe, thrifting is a great way to pick up a few pieces to get started.

If looking at clothing sizes and the thought of shopping for a new wardrobe feels overwhelming, you might consider asking a clinician on your treatment team to nominate you for The Garment Project, a nonprofit designed to provide new tag-less, size-less clothing for free to people in different stages of recovery from an ED. For more information, check out thegarmentproject.org.

Lastly, create a "friendly closet" that has you choosing clothes that make you feel good in them and about yourself, and rid your closet of items that don't do that. "Comfort" is key. *Being comfortable is not some commitment to a new size, forever and ever. You are allowed to be comfortable today without it saying anything about tomorrow.* Where you will "land" in your recovery, physically and psychologically, is yet to be discovered. This is the antithesis of the ED's ethos of "controlling your body in all ways." We invite you to trust your body in all ways.

Be patient. Be kind. Be comfortable.

Tips for Shopping Success

1. Shop when you are calm, well-rested, hydrated, and fed.

2. Consider speaking to your therapist about how to navigate this task successfully.

3. Take time to imagine how it will go. Will it be fun, or are you nervous and worried about becoming overwhelmed? If you imagine the latter, consider shopping online first so you can try clothes on in the comfort of your own home.

4. Take stock of what you currently have in your closet and drawers. What fits and has room for growth if further weight gain is needed? What doesn't fit?

5. Anything that doesn't fit needs to go. Keeping any clothing item that is too small only fuels the ED, as these are "sick" clothes that won't allow you to continue to move forward in your recovery.

6. Do not hand down the clothes that don't fit to friends or family. This will lead you to feel jealous that others get to be that weight, yet you can't. Donate them. You should never have to see those clothes again!

7. During the recovery process, you may be highly sensitive to the feeling of the waistband in your clothing. Consider buying stretchy, breathable, and loose pants instead of jeans. Breezy dresses without a waistline will feel better than form-fitting ones. There are many fashionable options for clothes that can help you feel more comfortable during this phase.

8. Remember, you will eventually be able to wear tighter clothing and feel comfortable in them, though this will take time.

9. Consider buying a few weight-neutral options as well—fun socks, a new necklace, or a hat, which you can get excited about without focusing on size.

10. Don't look at sizes. Sizes vary greatly and don't mean anything! Perhaps someone can help bring you clothes, and you can try them on without looking at the sizes.

Reduce Body Checking Behaviors

"Body checking" is a term used to describe an obsessive scrutiny toward parts of one's body to see if they have changed in any way. A person might pinch or pull their skin, stare at their reflection, compare old photos, keep "progress photos," and try on old clothes to see if they still fit.

Scrutiny breeds dissatisfaction. It increases anxiety, depression, and feelings of diminished control regarding shape and weight. If we're looking for flaws, we're going to find them. Body checking can increase stress and anxiety and detracts from confidence and a state of peace. Small shifts our bodies can be accompanied by changes in mood, which can subsequently cause a desire to act on ED symptomatology. Body checking increases one's risk for an ED.[4]

The first step in reducing body checking is to become aware of its frequency. Being aware of body checking behaviors can be helpful in appreciating how often you are harboring a negative narrative about yourself, which draws attention to a behavior you can start to shift. If you see mirrors as a weapon versus a tool (they hurt, not help), consider as a temporary measure removing them or covering them with a cloth—or with affirmations. The goal would be to use the practice of "habit reversal" to interrupt the behavior of body checking.[5] This means interrupting the behavior before it starts and replacing it with something equally appealing, which will vary by person.

Step 1: Awareness

When are you body checking?

Where are you body checking (at home/at work)?

How are you body checking (photos, using old clothes, while on Zoom calls)?

Which parts of the day do you find you do this the most?

Step 2: What's triggering this for you?

Step 3: Can you brainstorm alternative coping mechanisms?

Step 4: Take action! Which areas can you adjust?

For example:

Can you remove or cover mirrors?

Can you hide your "self-view" during virtual meetings?

Can you get rid of old clothes that you are body checking against?

Can you delete old "progress photos" that you are comparing your current body to?

Ditch the Scale

Another form of body checking is self-weighing. Most would agree that weighing yourself repeatedly is obsessive and not likely to help improve your body image. Multiple weight checks reflect only the daily fluctuations of fluids, food, stool, salt, and more—all the while causing you to feel stressed, anxious, and reactive about what the number on the scale says. And what's in a number anyway? Tying morality to a number ("I'm good if my weight is in the 'desired' range, and 'bad' if it's in the undesired range") creates a very fragile sense of self-confidence and self-worth.

Self-weighing can also negatively affect mood. When a person sees the number on the scale increase, there is often a negative response. "I could be having a great day, but if the scale is up, it ruins my day," one client said. Detaching your worth from the number on the scale is important.

Note that ongoing weight checks might be important for those who are medically compromised. This is best determined by your medical team in consideration of what is best for your care. If weight checks are required by your treatment team and going into the office solely to have your weight checked feels burdensome, you might consider utilizing a numberless scale such as the MyClearStep scale or Blind Weight, which allow you to step on a numberless scale that transmits the data directly to your team.

Like, Unfollow, Follow . . .

Social media sites like Instagram and TikTok have received a lot of scrutiny over the years for negatively impacting the mental health of their users—and rightfully so. A recent study at Griffith University in Australia showed that watching just seven minutes of "beauty content" in one session on TikTok and Instagram is enough for people to experience significant shame and anxiety about their appearance.[6] Consider the following social media tips for reducing body image distress.

- Consider who you are following and why. Are the "experts" you are trusting credentialed?

- Unfollow triggering influencers on your social media! Studies show that even briefly viewing #fitspo #thinspo (fitness and weight loss images/influencers) can negatively affect body image.

- Follow influencers with diverse body shapes and sizes, from diverse racial and ethnic backgrounds. Here, social media can be an ally. Look for influencers who speak out against body-shaming.

- Diversify your feed to include other interests: sports, hobbies, pets, travel, crafts, and people who align with your interests and values.

- Set a timer for social media apps on your phone (look in your phone's settings for this option) to limit social media use.

- Turn off notifications for apps you are trying to use less.

- Consider socializing in real life (make a date with a friend or a family member to provide authentic connection).

Separate Bad Body Image Feelings from Your Food

One of the most important tenets of ED work is to learn to separate your feelings from your food intake. Should a bad body image day strike, it's important to eat and follow your meal plan *anyway*. This is hard! But as you do the work and discover that underneath the bad body image day is a feeling (fear? stress? anger?), it becomes easier to nourish yourself. As your mindset gets more recovery oriented, you might begin to feel more committed to the meal plan for benefits you discover along the way. "My brain fog has lifted" or "I can finally keep up with my kids" or "I actually have energy." These discoveries reinforce eating, even when it's hard. Keeping body image distress separate from whether you eat or not is key to navigating a successful recovery.

Build a Life Outside the Identification with Your Body

Creating a life outside your ED is key to moving away from the focus on your body. Building community with friends, participating in sports, socializing, volunteering, taking classes, going back to work, or going to meetups can help you shift away from the preoccupation you might have with your body. Cameron was a college student who valued how her brain came back online as she became better nourished. She was studying psychology and languages and loved writing. She felt less foggy, more centered, and less stressed about her food and body when better nourished. She had more interests and could sleep better. "The strength of my brain helps me keep up the strength of my body," she explained. This was a constant reminder to her that, "I do not want my eating disorder."

Building a life can be hard for people. Where can you start? Being medically stable is an important step. Being fully nourished to access your full self is important, too. You can then begin to find activities that might interest you. A new business? A hobby? Dating? Sometimes, it starts with signing up for a class, or starting a new job. This is one of the most exciting parts of therapy and ED treatment: discovering what comes next!

CHAPTER 19

"I need you to know THIS!" (For Family and Friends in My Life)

IN A DIET-OBSESSED, "wellness-infused" world, nuances of language can cause harm to individuals in ED recovery. Diet culture is so pervasive that it becomes almost shocking to see someone *actually* eating regular and consistent meals. There are often comments about what people are eating, about people's bodies (without their consent) and about burning off calories to lose weight. These comments cause harm to those who are in ED recovery and, really, to anyone! Many of your loved ones may have spent a lifetime dieting and might still be struggling with their own relationship with weight, food, and body. In this chapter, we will offer guidance for your family, friends, and loved ones in the areas of food, body, and exercise.

FOOD

"I need to eat 3 meals and 2 or 3 snacks."

Your meal plan is essential for recovery. Yet, we often hear how those around you might observe and comment on what you are eating.

"You're eating again?"

"You need *all* that?"

"I could never eat that. I would gain so much weight."

"How do you eat so much? Where do you put it?"

"I am just too full, but you go ahead."

"Don't you get full?"

These comments immediately create a comparison that is challenging for the ED, causing it to want you to eat less, compensate, or give up altogether. You might want to advise friends and relatives in advance that they just shouldn't say anything about your food—unless it is a neutral comment.

"Pass the ketchup, please."

"Is this the right temperature?"

"Do you like what I made tonight?"

They can also speak encouragingly.

"I am here for you."

"How can I help? What do you need?"

"Do you need help shopping?"

"Can I help set the table?"

"Would it be helpful if I ate this meal with you?"

"Can I cook you something?"

Comments about the volume of food make the person with an ED feel like they are eating too much. What is more likely, though, is that the person in recovery is following the recommendations from their treatment team. For example, seemingly harmless comments like "Oh, I'm so full!" or "That dessert looks delicious but I really shouldn't" from a loved one can make the person with an ED feel ashamed about finishing their plate of food. It becomes hard for the person in recovery to keep moving forward. Don't let comments derail your recovery! It's important you do what is best for you. Surround yourself with people who respect your needs and wishes.

It can be helpful to brainstorm with your family members what conversation topics are positive to talk about and which ones to avoid. This helps the home become a place of safety in the face of an ED—a safe zone, protected from the messages you are inundated with in the outside world. This will also give your family a chance to talk about other things: politics, sports, work, school, and relationships. For that reason, it can be helpful to decide on ground rules for family time conversation.

Safe topics: work, travel, friends

Topics to avoid: weight, dieting, good/bad foods, other people's weight, health issues

Mealtimes work best when there is fun, light conversation.

"It's triggering to me when you don't eat."

Many of our patients report that a loved one has an ED. The loved one tries to support them but doesn't model balanced eating themselves. This is incredibly challenging and confusing for individuals who are working hard to fight against diet messaging, to eat more regularly, and to recover. Seeing a loved one's ED displayed without any attempt to rein it in often angers our patients and doesn't feel fair.

We try to remind our patients, "We are treating *you*," and while it's triggering and restricting for your loved one to be avoiding meals, it's important for you to continue to do what's best for *you*. Remember: You can provide a direct and pointed invitation to your loved one, such as, "Will you join me for lunch?"

Setting a Boundary

If your loved one is still not listening to your requests, it might be time to set a firm boundary. Saying no can feel avoidant but is often protective of your recovery. The boundary you set might be only temporary, until you feel strong enough in your recovery to withstand what comes your way.

Examples

- A boundary might be saying no to spending Thanksgiving with a family member who is not able to join you for meals or who can't stop talking about their diet.
- You might say no to a vacation getaway with a partner who is overly focused on their body and on having six-pack abs.
- You might break up with someone because they are obsessed with every single thing they put into their mouth, count calories, and do all the things you have worked so hard to *stop* doing.
- You might say no to having a certain grandparent watch your kids, when you hear how they talk about food and weight in front of your children, despite being asked to stop.

"I don't want to hear about your diet."

Talking about diets, dieting, and "bad" foods in front of someone with an ED is not advised under any circumstances. Talking about "cutting carbs" or "avoiding saturated fats" could make the person in recovery feel bad about eating what's on their plate. Comments about wanting to avoid desserts are likely to make the individual feel guilty about eating those foods, reinforcing the notion that there are "bad foods" out there. Hearing a loved one say that "they aren't going to eat much at dinner because they ate *way too much* at lunch" aligns with the ED's desire to intellectually adjust one's diet rather than let their body naturally decide, which is something they will need to learn to do. These types of comments make it even harder to eat than it already is. You might need to ask family members and loved ones whether they can join you in your journey to food acceptance.

Family functions are notorious for weight and diet conversation. It would not be surprising to attend a family function with your extended family and find your aunt Ramona chatting in the corner about how she lost some number of pounds by cutting out carbohydrates, white flour, and sugar. This will likely be triggering as you seek to reestablish your relationship with food. Hearing this, even from a distant relative, could make you ponder whether you should also avoid these foods (please don't!) or if there is something wrong with you for eating these foods (all food is good food!). The ED also gets jealous hearing about others "getting" to lose weight while you are actively fighting back against these tough concepts.

Here, you might pull your family member aside privately in the moment and share with them however much you want to about what's going on for you. You might explain why what they are talking about is difficult for you or your philosophy around that kind of language. It's hard to advocate for yourself, but it's important—this can be a pivotal teachable moment for this person.

Remember, you don't have to go at it alone. Your treatment team will work with you on strategies to field these messages about food, weight, and shape. The reality is that someone, somewhere will always be talking about their new diet or desire to lose weight. Therefore, an important aspect of recovery is to build armor to shield against these comments so they don't shake you as much. Think: "What's right for *me*?" For you to be healthy, you need to eat a balanced plate that contains all food groups, to not skip meals, and to have your snacks. Some of you need to gain weight, restore vital signs and hormonal balance. If you are feeling confused about recovery, you can always revisit your "whys for recovery" (page 119).

"I will not do a cleanse with you."

Dieting is harmful for recovery. It's possible your loved one, with whom you or your ED might have dieted in the past, still has not received the memo: detox programs, cleanses, diets, and fasts are not part of your recovery plans. Dieting for even a few days will activate body image distress and a desire to change your body, which can diminish you emotionally and physically.

You will likely have to explain your recovery goals. For example, "To protect my recovery, I have committed to eating regular, full meals, that contain all food groups, three times a day, plus snacks. This helps to keep my mind clear, prevent me from bingeing, and obsessing about food so much. A cleanse just puts me on that merry-go-round with food and doesn't help support me with my recovery goals. If anything, it would carry me further away from them."

"Please don't compliment my body."

When a loved one makes what seems like a benign comment to someone with an ED—"You look great!" or "You look healthy!"—the ED might hear this as, "Oh, so everyone thinks I look bad now." Comments that are meant to be encouraging and celebratory of someone's hard work in recovery such as, "You look so much better than you used to," make someone in recovery feel very aware that their body looks different to the person making the comment. It makes the person with the ED uncomfortable with their new body (they think: "Everyone can see I look different now"), and this can make the person want to give up rather than keep going.

The best compliments are ones that notice someone's mood, energy, or the coloring in someone's eyes or face. For example, "You seem so much more energetic now." That might be tricky, too, if someone isn't feeling as you have described. As The Body Positive's Connie Sobczak explains, "For me, I'll say to someone, 'Your energy is so radiant, how are you doing? What's going on in your life?' But someone might be having a bad day and feel like they're not that radiant. Let's just start in on the conversation without having to comment on each other in any way, shape, or form."

We recommend that loved ones avoid commenting on someone's body at all. If someone loses weight, and you compliment them, they tend not to feel great when they gain the weight back (which statistically is more than likely to occur). "You look thin" turns into, "Did I not look thin before?" or "Why are you scrutinizing my body?" We might feel sadness or insecurity when the compliment doesn't come next time.

Talking about other people's bodies and praising weight loss can be interpreted by the person with an ED (or by someone who is susceptible) as "I should lose weight so I look good." Similarly, hearing a discussion about someone's recent weight loss and "how great they look" reinforces that being thin is valued and praised. Making a comment that someone in your community "got so much bigger" in front of someone in ED recovery is fatphobic and highlights that you notice and disapprove of these changes. This will terrify the person in ED recovery, causing them to worry, "What if I get bigger, what will everyone think of me then?"

Size acceptance is a hallmark of treatment, but comments like this can undo progress. Finally, when members of your inner circle comment on their own bodies, it communicates to the person in recovery that if *they* are critical of *their* own body, how and why could they ever accept yours?

"I might look okay, but many days I am not."

In other words, "Just because my body looks okay to you, *please understand and respect* that I am struggling on the inside."

We can't tell by size who is struggling or the degree to which someone is struggling. This is one of the ED stereotypes that many activists and professionals are trying to break: Those in larger bodies often face weight stigma, receive less support, experience more criticism, have less access to services, and receive less care than those in smaller bodies. One's relationship with food and body is not something you can accurately judge by outward physical appearance. Loved ones should not assume those struggling "are better now" because of what they see physically.

"Please don't comment on my clothing."

It's possible you might need different clothing sizes if you have experienced physical changes. This might be stressful, and it requires time and acceptance that you need new clothing. There might be times when you are wearing old clothing that is too small or phases in which you have bought some newer clothing, but only a few pieces, which you wear regularly.

You might need to remind loved ones that you need some peace and space to navigate these changes. Comments that clothing "looks tight" or inquiries such as, "Why are you wearing the same clothing over and over again?" will likely remind you that you feel unsettled in this new space. You will need to remind loved ones not to make comments about clothing.

"Don't talk about burning calories."

It's important to observe how those around you talk about exercise. Exercising to burn calories, lose weight, or alter one's appearance creates an unhealthy relationship with movement. Linking exercise to food intake in any way—"I ate too much today, I have to work out"—sends the message that we need to compensate with exercise for food consumed. Of course, we are working on moving joyfully, listening to our body, and NOT moving to burn calories. Messages associated with a diet mindset are very unhelpful for those in recovery.

"I don't need to earn my dessert."

Let's not link one's food intake to whether or not someone exercised that day. Your body is very active—from digestion to brain function to respiration—and needs food to survive. Exercise makes up only a small part of an individual's energy expenditure, as we learned in chapter 13. Regardless of whether you went to the gym or played sports, your body has the ability to digest and process dessert, or anything else you decide to eat. The body is amazing that way. But linking the two increases feelings of guilt and shame around movement and desserts (or whichever food you want to "burn off"). The body is always working at digestion; it's a twenty-four-hour process. There is no need to run or bike or go to the gym afterward. Loved ones should aim to catch themselves before linking food and movement this way, right along with you!

"Can you join me this week in taking a rest day?"

Watching a loved one prioritize movement above all else sends the message that one's appearance and body are the most important things. When someone trains through injury, or trains through important deadlines, events, or social engagements, it sends the message that exercise is more important than health, work, and socialization.

This is triggering for an individual going through recovery, since they are usually working on their relationship with movement. This often includes taking at least one rest day per week, if not more. The ED does not *want* to rest, but you are trying to follow guidelines so the body can recover, muscles can repair and grow, and inflammation can subside. But when someone else is ignoring those recommendations, the ED gets jealous. (*Wait, if they can do that, why can't I?*) Remember: Copying unhealthy behaviors will not help you recover!

For loved ones, recognize how tempting, confusing, and challenging these observations are for someone in recovery. The person who is in recovery might ask their loved one directly, "Can you join me this week when I take my rest day?" This will convey the message that rest is something that should be prioritized.

"You might miss my eating disorder."

As you get better and say goodbye to many of the ED behaviors, it's possible your loved one might miss some of those behaviors. Maybe you used to connect around some of these behaviors, such as running, bingeing, or dieting. Maybe they miss their binge-buddy, exercise partner, or food-focused friend. Have compassion, and also recognize that this is their path to figure out. Let them know it's true that how you approach meals or exercise is different in recovery, and know there are many ways to connect to others outside of meals and exercise.

"Thank you."

An ED is not easy. It can be demanding, erratic, and often challenging to support. It's okay to let your loved one know you are grateful to them for listening to this long list of requests and for considering making changes in their language and actions. Thanking them for their support, and for being there throughout your journey, is positive reinforcement. Remember: You don't ever have to apologize for your illness. Apologizing implies you have done something wrong. Being sick is not something you did wrong or on purpose. But you can acknowledge that your illness has been hard for others and support them right back by asking if they have everything *they* need. Do you have someone to talk to? Do you have a way to take care of yourself during this stressful time in our lives?

While it's challenging to share these comments, requests, and boundaries with loved ones, doing so will ultimately support your recovery. Creating safety in your home, especially in the early stages, is important for quieting the ED. As you progress further along in recovery, it will be easier to weather the challenges that come up and practice building resiliency. Once you are on more stable ground, challenges will be easier for you to navigate. We promise.

CHAPTER 20

Normal Eating

HERE YOU ARE. You've spent countless hours in ED appointments and worked incredibly hard to get to this point. You might even be wondering if you need to continue going to your appointments. You're eating regular meals and snacks that are adequate and satisfying. And that ED voice that used to run the show? It's quiet, sometimes barely noticeable. If this resonates with you, welcome to the final stages of ED treatment. This is where it gets good. This is where you get your life back and *you* get to be in the driver's seat. That said, you're not done yet. There's still work to do in this last phase of treatment.

You've been following the Plate-by-Plate Approach®, eating 3 meals and 2 or 3 snacks per day and finishing 100 percent of your plate. Nice work! Now it's time to shake things up as you work toward normal eating. At this point the meals and snacks should feel doable, and your body will have adjusted to the volume of food so that you no longer feel overly full, bloated, constipated, etc. Those symptoms described in chapters 2 and 11 may still come and go in waves or at completely unexpected times, which is normal. But these symptoms should now be occurring much less frequently. In the meantime, you have gained tools to help talk back to the ED voice when it sneaks back in. And you feel ready to take this next step toward "normal eating" so that you can accomplish the following.

- Regain a sense of normalcy around eating.
- Learn to trust your body to guide your eating choices rather than rely

on this book or your treatment team to tell you what, when, and how to eat.

- Finally, reclaim food freedom and become a fearless eater.

What Is Normal Eating?

Our goal during this process is to teach you how to eat normally again. This includes learning to respond to your hunger cues so you can eat when you are hungry and stop when you are full. Ellyn Satter, MS, RD, an internationally recognized expert on feeding and eating, describes the following characteristics of "normal" eating.[1]

- Going to the table hungry and eating until you are satisfied
- Being able to choose food you like, eat it, and truly get enough of it—not stopping because you think you should
- Being able to give some thought to your food selection so you get nutritious food, but not being so wary and restrictive that you miss out on enjoyable food
- Giving yourself permission to eat sometimes because you are happy, sad, or bored, or just because it feels good
- Eating mostly 3 meals a day, or 4 or 5, or choosing to munch along the way
- Leaving some cookies on the plate because you know you can have some again tomorrow, or eating more now because they taste so wonderful
- Overeating at times, feeling stuffed and uncomfortable
- Undereating at times and wishing you had more
- Trusting your body to make up for your mistakes in eating
- Letting eating consume some of your time and attention but keeping its place as only one important area of your life

In short, normal eating is flexible. It varies in response to your hunger, your schedule, your proximity to food, and your feelings. It can take a long time for those who have battled EDs to reach that level of normalcy around eating. You might first see glimmers of it as you begin to spontaneously graze or pick at food between meals. These are signs that you are shifting away from rigidity and obsessiveness and moving toward fearless eating. It can take a long time for those behaviors to emerge, and they are usually a great indicator that you are heading in the right direction.

How Do I Know When I'm Ready for This Step?

You are ready to take the next step when you:

- consistently maintain medical stability, including weight and vital signs (REQUIRED),
- are getting regular periods (biological females, not including those in perimenopause or menopause),
- enjoy food again,
- experience cravings for foods you used to love and actually eat,
- can eat spontaneously (i.e., grabbing a few pieces of chocolate after dinner because it "sounds good"),
- are more flexible with food, eating what is served without fear,
- can eat out at a restaurant without heightened anxiety or stress.

Maintaining medical stability means you are physically in a safe and healthy place. At that stable place, your heart and brain are sufficiently nourished. Your metabolism has probably normalized, allowing you to correctly understand your hunger and satiety cues. By this point, your anxiety around food is generally greatly reduced. If you remain unstable, you are likely not ready for this next step in treatment.

If you are stable physically and have not had a period, please speak to your treatment team to determine if you are ready for this next step. Skipped periods may be a lingering sign that your energy balance is not yet stable. Perhaps you are exercising too much, not eating enough, or not consuming enough dietary fats. In those cases, you might want to wait to make changes to meals. Or your weight and mindset may be in a great place, but your menstrual cycles and hormone levels will need time to return. Normalized menstrual cycles can take up to six months after achieving weight restoration.[2] Your physician can do lab work to check current estradiol levels, which indicate how close you are to getting your period back. If you are in a good place mentally and you are exhibiting some of the signs of normal eating (see page 272), it's possible to take this next step despite amenorrhea. For biological males, you can use vital signs, testosterone levels, and psychological mindset to determine whether you are ready.

Gaining Confidence

In addition to medical stability, another important aspect of transitioning to normal eating is gauging whether the ED still has a hold over you and to what degree. You may want to consider the following.

- Are you confident that you can finish meals and obtain adequate nutrition from all meals and snacks?

- Are you eating a wide variety of foods (including those that were previously challenging)?

- Can you eat confidently in a wide variety of settings (e.g., restaurants, family's and friends' houses, fast-food establishments, takeout, potluck-style meals, parties, and so on)?

If you answered no to any of these questions, you may want to continue eating in a more structured way until you can answer yes to all the questions.

**What to Do If the Eating Disorder
Still Has a Firm Grip on You**

Here are some things to consider if you continue to experience difficulty with an ED.

1. Are you really at the right weight? Have your team reassess your weight goals. The treatment goals for weight provided by your team early on might need to be adjusted.

2. Can you work on more food exposure? If you are struggling, you might need to work on increasing exposure to challenging foods. A renewed focus on increasing variety will help you become more flexible with food.

3. Set small, achievable goals such as "eating one meal at a restaurant" or "trying one new food" this weekend.

4. Practice choosing "yummy" foods. Try going to a restaurant, sitting with the menu, and ordering what sounds good to you rather than ordering what is "safe" or what you think you "should eat." Mastering these skills paves the way for normal eating.

Greater Comfort around Food

Once you are in a physically healthy place, you may begin to crave certain foods. Suddenly, you are in the kitchen making your grandma's casserole recipe that you once swore you'd never eat again because of the "scary" ingredients. Your birthday rolls around and instead of stressing over whether you'll be able to eat a bite of birthday cake, you are excited to eat it, and may even eat a second slice because it's so good. Going to a restaurant is no longer a reason for fear and anxiety; instead, you thrill at the prospect of trying new foods. During this stage, you finally begin to feel comfortable ordering from a menu, eating with others, and exploring food again. This is the reward that comes from all your hard work in earlier stages of treatment.

By this time, you have likely become so used to "exposure, exposure, exposure" that all foods become fair game. You can finally taste the flavors in food without feeling stressed and can explore different food choices without the fear that those foods are going to make you unhealthy. Somewhere along the way it happened: You started to like food again!

You may have also started eating spontaneously again. For example, you try a bite of your partner's entrée at a restaurant one night, something you never would have done before because that would have been "extra." Or you ate a brownie at work because someone brought them in to share, even though you had already eaten a morning snack. You may start to graze, such as grabbing a handful of pretzels before dinner or taking some nuts that were in a bowl on the counter after lunch. These new behaviors are often shocking and signal that you are moving forward. You may secretly wonder, is this okay? The answer is an unqualified yes. This is part of the process of returning to normal eating.

Flexibility around food generally increases during this time. Flexibility means you are eating different foods each day—different breakfasts, lunches, dinners, and snacks—and your eating may follow a less specific pattern. Sudden meal changes that result from running out of something or being unable to go to the store don't rattle you as they did before. For example, if you planned on making a turkey sandwich for lunch only to realize that the turkey meat has expired, you're able to quickly shift and make yourself a salami sandwich instead. If a friend invites you to their house for dinner, you no longer stress about what's being served.

You may still experience body image concerns, but at this point you find that those concerns no longer drive your actions around food. While you may feel dissatisfied with your body, you are generally able to keep it from affecting your food intake.

Testing the Waters

To decide if you are ready for this next step, some (if not all) of the behaviors previously discussed should be present, along with medical stabilization. Spontaneous eating, even if it happens only once or twice, demonstrates that you are moving in the right direction. Taking a second helping or adding something to your meal means that you are no longer adhering to rigid food rules. Honoring food cravings demonstrates an interest in food again. These behaviors will happen naturally, *when you are ready*. Once these positive behaviors occur, you can safely work toward a more flexible and normal style of eating.

Small tests, whether it's going to a new restaurant, traveling, or trying a new recipe, are all experiences that provide you with information about your recovery. Can you be successful under those circumstances? Did you learn something new about your lingering food fears from the experiment? Though it has been exhausting to get to this point, you are now more resilient and are likely to be more capable of getting back on track should you get derailed. Unlike the beginning of treatment, you can now instantly recognize the warning signs that something is off, and you have the tools to steer yourself back to the right path.

Identifying and Responding to Hunger Cues

If you are ready to progress to normal eating, you must learn to understand your hunger and satiety cues. In the earlier stages of treatment, it is very common for an individual with an ED to say they just don't feel any hunger or fullness cues: "I only feel full; I never feel hungry." This is partly due to the physiological changes that occur during the refeeding process, plus the high volume of food required for those in need of weight gain. It can also occur when someone goes from chaotic eating and dieting to a more stabilized meal plan. Even in the absence of needing to gain weight, some are surprised at how often they have to eat to stabilize their ED. Anxiety around food can also inhibit a person's hunger levels. Being at a stable weight and on a regular schedule of meals allows you to get in touch with your body again. However, it may still be possible that you do not recognize these cues.

You may be used to feeling extreme hunger (from periods of food restriction) and have come to perceive that as "normal" hunger. Alternatively, you may be very sensitive to hunger and perceive a small pang of hunger as a sign that you aren't eating enough. We expect that you will feel hungry prior to meals and snacks; that is a signal that it's nearing time to eat. Fluctuating levels of hunger are completely normal and should occur regularly throughout the day. Feeling full is normal and usually passes thirty to sixty minutes after a meal.

To master this part, you can begin to track your hunger and fullness levels throughout the day. You can rate these cues on a scale of 1 to 10, with 1 being starving and 10 being extremely full, using the hunger meter.[3] Initially, you may struggle to decipher what your body is feeling. But with practice, you will begin to understand your hunger and fullness cues. You will compare how you felt at breakfast to how you felt at lunch, and again at dinner. And slowly, you will be reacquainted with your appetite.

It's good to arrive at a meal or a snack with "manageable hunger," which would be a level 3 or 4. Ideally, you are hungry, but not starving. If your hunger level reaches a 1 on the hunger scale before the meal, that is a clear sign that you didn't eat enough at the last meal or snack, or perhaps you waited too long to eat this next meal. It's then easy to bypass your body's natural stopping place at this meal. Become curious rather than judgmental if this happens. Was my meal too small? Did I not eat enough of a snack? After a meal, a good stopping point for fullness might be a 6 or 7. As you reach toward a 9 or 10, you'll begin to feel uncomfortably full. Following a regular schedule, in which you continue to eat every 3 to 4 hours, will help keep your blood sugar stable and stimulate your appetite while preventing hunger from becoming extreme.

This part of treatment is more of an art than a science. It takes time, practice, and a lot of patience. It will be bumpy, scary, and awkward, but in time it will lead you to be a truly normal eater.

Meal Guidelines for Normal Eating

As you transition to normal eating, follow these rough guidelines so that the ED doesn't lead you astray.

Stick to a schedule of 3 meals and 2 or 3 snacks, where all food groups are present. Many think that once at this stage they can abandon a meal schedule and the guidelines provided. This is not recommended. Meals and snacks should be spaced no more than three hours apart. This is your road map and will help you reconnect with your intuitive hunger and fullness cues. It also won't change—in fact, we recommend this meal structure for most people, whether or not they are recovering from an ED. Eating regularly keeps blood sugar levels stable throughout the day, keeps hunger in the desired range (preventing over- and undereating), and improves energy and concentration.

Allow flexibility with how much you "have to" finish at mealtime. Before, you were expected to eat 100 percent of food on the plate. Now, you can check in with your body before, during, and after the meal to decide how much you need to eat. You can consider your level of hunger or fullness after you have completed about 75 percent of your plate (less than that may signal food restriction). Are you satisfied? Still hungry? Do you want more? How does your stomach feel? If you decide you are genuinely satisfied, you can stop eating at this point. This is especially helpful for restaurant meals, which might be larger portions than you might serve at home, so completing 100 percent of a meal is less intuitive. Interestingly, most of the time, individuals continue to eat 100 percent of their plates even once granted this new freedom, because they are truly hungry and because the food *tastes* good. This shift may take you by surprise. It's so different from what you have become accustomed to during this process. But allowing yourself to leave behind some food or have second helpings if you wish strengthens your own intuition around food.

Those who eat 75 percent at one meal and stop there should be aware that they may be hungrier at the next meal. They might therefore eat 125 percent at the next meal, taking seconds. Being able to have more at the next meal is an important factor to consider when evaluating if you are ready to take a step toward normal eating: Can you have *more* than what's on your plate if you are still hungry? This can be a very challenging process and will take practice. You will likely second-guess yourself: "Did I eat too much?" "Do I still need more?" There is more room for interpretation in this phase than before, when meals needed to be completed 100 percent. In time, however, you will make your way toward eating intuitively and normally.

Be spontaneous. This is the first time in treatment that you decide how much you need, which can be scary. Keep an open mind while navigating this step. If you want to eat something spontaneously between meals and snacks (e.g., a cookie or an apple), allow yourself to have it and continue to the next scheduled meal or snack as usual. You might find that this additional food has little to no impact on your appetite at the next meal or you might find that you are fuller and unable to finish the next meal or snack. Either way, make room for this spontaneity and try not to compensate at the next meal.

Eat a minimum of 75 percent at the next meal or snack. If you are too full because you had that extra food item, make a point to eat 75 percent anyway. That way there's no risk of the ED creeping back into mealtime. Along the way, you will learn what feels good to your body in terms of spontaneous snacking and how that affects mealtime.

Don't expect perfection. This is the beginning of a new period of trial and error with food. You may get it "right" some of the time and "wrong" at others. That's okay. The main goal is to explore hunger and fullness cues again and to practice as you learn how to eat *normally*.

As this process continues, allow yourself to plan meals and snacks based on foods you used to love and may have restricted in earlier stages of treatment. For example, if you used to love a particular brand of ice cream, go get a scoop or two. If you have been hesitant to try pepperoni pizza, order delivery! The key here is to normalize everything while learning to become an adventurous eater again.

Trouble Signs

As you embark on this new leg of the journey, here are some red flags to watch out for.

- You consistently eat only the bare minimum (75 percent) at meals and snacks. That is a sign you are not eating based on your intuition but are likely eating based on food rules the ED has created.

- Your food variety is narrowing and you consistently choose "safe" foods reminiscent of earlier stages of treatment.

- At medical check-ins, you are consistently losing weight.

- ED thoughts become louder and more frequent.

These red flags don't necessarily mean that you cannot move forward with this more normal way of eating. You might need to practice in a more limited way—for example, only at dinnertime. Sometimes, a more gradual approach is necessary for this transition to be successful and effective. Either way, good communication with your treatment team about the challenges you are facing is key. And while the end goal is to reestablish a healthy relationship with food, the path is usually not linear. It is important to continue working toward "normal" eating.

Closing Thoughts

If you have made it to this point, congratulations! You have done a tremendous amount of work. You have fought hard to get your life back, and you have saved yourself from the relentless grip of an ED. Eating "normally" again is a huge accomplishment and you should feel relieved to be here. And while you may have finished reading this book, remember that the Plate-by-Plate Approach® will always be a tool you can rely on to stay on track with food.

Recovery takes several months, if not years, to solidify. Don't be surprised if your recovery includes some ups and downs along the way. The difference now is that you have become more resilient in the face of obstacles and more committed to your recovery. And you know first-hand the dangers associated with taking your emotions out on your food and body. At some point, you will be truly free to eat however you want. Yet, you will always need to be vigilant about big changes in your diet.

Relapse can happen. What's important is that you now have the skills to stay ahead of the ED, to notice where it may hide, to be curious about changes in eating and exercise behaviors, and to "go back to what worked last" at any point should recovery shift to relapse. Hopefully, you will maintain a fully recovered life, made possible by all the effort you put toward treatment, and this ED will keep its place as only one difficult chapter of your otherwise healthy and happy life.

We salute you! You are a force to be reckoned with.

NOTES

Introduction

1. "Social and economic cost of eating disorders in the US," Deloitte Access Economics, July 2020, www2.deloitte.com/au/en/pages/economics/articles/social-economic-cost-eating-disorders-united-states.html.

2. J. Arcelus et al., "Mortality rates in patients with anorexia nervosa and other eating disorders: A meta-analysis of 36 studies," *Archives of General Psychiatry* 68, no. 7 (2011): 724–31.

3. J. I. Hudson et al., The prevalence and correlates of eating disorders in the National Comorbidity Survey Replication," *Biological Psychiatry* 61, no. 3 (February 2007): 348–58.

   S. A. Swanson, et al., "Prevalence and correlates of eating disorders in adolescents. Results from the national comorbidity survey replication adolescent supplement," *Archives of General Psychiatry* 68, no. 7 (July 2011): 714–23.

4. M. F. Flament et al., "Weight status and DSM-5 diagnoses of eating disorders in adolescents from the community," *Journal of the American Academy of Child and Adolescent Psychiatry* 54, no. 5 (May 2015): 403–11.

5. C. C. Simpson et al., "Calorie Counting and Fitness Tracking Technology: Associations with Eating Disorder Symptomatology," *Eating Behaviors* 26 (August 2017): 89–92.

   J. Linardon and M. Messer, "My fitness pal usage in men: Associations with eating disorder symptoms and psychosocial impairment," *Eating Behaviors* 33 (April 2019): 13–17.

   C. A. Levinson et al., "My Fitness Pal calorie tracker usage in the eating disorders," *Eating Behaviors* 27 (December 2017): 14–16.

   M. Messer et al., "Using an app to count calories: Motives, perceptions, and connections to thinness- and muscularity-oriented disordered eating," *Eating Behaviors* 43 (December 2021): 101568.

Chapter 1

1. Z. Nikniaz et al., "A systematic review and meta-analysis of the prevalence and odds of eating disorders in patients with celiac disease and vice-versa," *International Journal of Eating Disorders* 54, no. 9 (September 2021): 1563–74.

    J. E. Peters et al., "Prevalence of disordered eating in adults with gastrointestinal disorders: A systematic review," *Neurogastroenterology & Motility* 34, no. 2 (October 2021): e14278.

2. K. M. Culbert et al., "Research Review: What we have learned about the causes of eating disorders – a synthesis of sociocultural, psychological, and biological research," *Journal of Child Psychology and Psychiatry* 56, no. 11 (June 2015): 1141–64.

3. E. Stice and M. J. V. Ryzin, "A Prospective Test of the Temporal Sequencing of Risk Factor Emergence in the Dual Pathway Model of Eating Disorders," *Journal of Abnormal Psychology* 128, no. 2 (February 2019): 119–28.

4. L. Smolak, "Body image development in childhood," in T. Cash and L. Smolak, eds., *Body Image: A Handbook of Science, Practice, and Prevention*, 2nd edition (New York: The Guilford Press, 2012).

5. A. E. Field et al., "Relation between dieting and weight change among preadolescents and adolescents," *Pediatrics* 112, no. 4 (October 2003): 900–6.

6. K. H. Pietiläinen et al., "Does dieting make you fat? A twin study," *International Journal of Obesity* 36, no. 3 (March 2012): 456–64.

7. N. H. Golden et al., "Preventing Obesity and Eating Disorders in Adolescents," *Pediatrics* 138, no. 3 (September 2016): e20161649.

8. Ibid.

9. M. Maine, interview by C. Cortese, ED Matters, January 25, 2021, audio, podcasts.apple.com/ie/podcast/episode-225-dr-margo-maine-eating-disorders-in-midlife/id1173632000?i=1000506472769.

10. "Breast Cancer Facts and Statistics," Breastcancer.org, January 18, 2023, breastcancer.org/facts-statistics.

11. M. Zayed and J. P. Garry, "Geriatric Anorexia Nervosa," *Journal of the American Board of Family Medicine* 30, no. 5 (September 2017): 666–69.

12. A. Hilbert et al., "How frequent are eating disturbances in the population? Norms of the eating disorder examination-questionnaire," *PLoS One* 7, no. 1 (2012): e29125.

13. C. V. Wiseman et al., "Changing patterns of hospitalization in eating disorder patients," *International Journal of Eating Disorders* 30, no. 1 (July 2001): 69–74.

14. American Psychiatric Association, *Diagnostic and Statistical Manual of Mental Disorders*, 5th Edition (Washington, DC: American Psychiatric Publishing, 2013).

15. S. F. Forman et al., "Predictors of outcome at 1 year in adolescents with DSM-5 restrictive eating disorders: report of the national eating disorders quality improvement collaborative," *Journal of Adolescent Health* 55, no. 6 (December 2014): 750–56.

16. G. A. Kennedy et al., "History of overweight/obesity as predictor of care received at 1-year follow-up in adolescents with anorexia nervosa or atypical anorexia nervosa," *Journal of Adolescent Health* 60, no. 6 (June 2017): 674–79.

    J. Lebow et al., "Prevalence of a history of overweight and obesity in adolescents with restrictive eating disorders," *Journal of Adolescent Health* 56, no. 1 (January 2015): 19–24.

17. "Binge Eating Disorder," National Eating Disorders Association, nationaleatingdisorders.org/learn/by-eating-disorder/bed.

18. K. R. Wells et al., "The Australian Institute of Sport (AIS) and National Eating Disorders Collaboration (NEDC) position statement on disordered eating in high performance sport," *British Journal of Sports Medicine* 54, no. 21 (November 2020): 1247–58.

19. Ibid.

20. P. E. Mosley, "Bigorexia: bodybuilding and muscle dysmorphia," *European Eating Disorders Review* 17, no. 3 (May 2009): 191–98.

21. S. B. Murray, PhD, and T. Baghurst, PhD, "Revisiting the Diagnostic Criteria for Muscle Dysmorphia," *Strength and Conditioning Journal* 35, no. 1 (February 2013): 69–74.

22. Ibid.

23. M. Fink et al., "When Is Patient Behavior Indicative of Avoidant Restrictive Food Intake Disorder (ARFID) Vs Reasonable Response to Digestive Disease?," *Clinical Gastroenterology and Hepatology* 20, no. 6 (June 2022): 1241–50.

    A. S. Day et al., "Food-related quality of life in adults with inflammatory bowel disease is associated with restrictive eating behaviour, disease activity and surgery: a prospective multicentre observational study," *Journal of Human Nutrition and Dietetics* 35, no. 1 (February 2022): 234–44.

24. F. Farag et al., "Avoidant/restrictive food intake disorder and autism spectrum disorder: clinical implications for assessment and management," *Developmental Medicine & Child Neurology* 64, no. 2 (February 2022): 176–82.

S. Yule et al., "Nutritional Deficiency Disease Secondary to ARFID Symptoms Associated with Autism and the Broad Autism Phenotype: A Qualitative Systematic Review of Case Reports and Case Series," *Journal of the Academy of Nutrition and Dietetics* 121, no. 3 (March 2021): 467–92.

25. D. Mitchison et al., "The prevalence and impact of eating disorder behaviours in Australian men," *Journal of Eating Disorders* 1, suppl. 1 (November 2013).

26. L. Cohn et al., "Including the excluded: Males and gender minorities in eating disorder prevention," *Eating Disorders: The Journal of Treatment & Prevention* 24, no. 1 (2016): 114–20.

27. M. Vo et al., "Eating Disorders in Adolescent and Young Adult Males: Presenting Characteristics," *Journal of Adolescent Health* 59, no. 4 (October 2016): 397–400.

28. T. Thomas, "NHS Hospital Admissions for Eating Disorders Rise Among Ethnic Minorities," *The Guardian*, October 18, 2020, theguardian.com/society/2020/oct/18/nhs-hospital-admissions-eating-disorders-rise-among-ethnic-minorities.

29. K. H. Gordon et al., "The Impact of Client Race on Clinician Detection of Eating Disorders," *Behavior Therapy* 37, no. 4 (December 2006): 319–25.

30. A. E. Becker et al., "Ethnicity and differential access to care for eating disorder symptoms," *International Journal of Eating Disorders* 33, no. 2 (March 2003): 205–12.

31. "Eating Disorder Statistics," National Association of Anorexia Nervosa and Associated Disorders, anad.org/eating-disorders-statistics.

32. L. L. Parker and J. A. Harriger, "Eating disorders and disordered eating behaviors in the LGBT population: a review of the literature," *International Journal of Eating Disorders* 16, no. 8 (October 2020): 51.

33. B. A. Jones et al., "Body dissatisfaction and disordered eating in trans people: A systematic review of the literature," *International Review of Psychiatry* 28, no. 1 (January 2016): 81–94.

34. T. A. Brown and P. K. Keel, "The impact of relationships on the association between sexual orientation and disordered eating in men," *International Journal of Eating Disorders* 45 (March 2012): 792–99.

35. A. R. Gordon et al., "Eating Disorders Among Transgender and Gender Non-binary People," in: J. M. Nagata et al., eds., *Eating Disorders in Boys and Men* (Edinburgh, Scotland: Springer, Cham, 2021).

E. W. Diemer et al., "Beyond the binary: Differences in eating disorder prevalence by gender identity in a transgender sample," *Transgender Health* 3, no. 1 (December 2018): 17–23.

36. M. Konstantinovsky, "If You Know Someone in the 2SLGBTQIA+ Community Who has an Eating Disorder, You'll Want to Read This," Equip, June 23, 2022, equip.health/articles/recovery/lgbtqia-support.

Chapter 2

1. D. Le Grange et al., "Early weight gain predicts outcome in two treatments for adolescent anorexia nervosa," *International Journal of Eating Disorders* 47, no. 2 (March 2014): 124–29.

2. "Global Weight Loss Products and Services Market Report 2021: The Business of Weight Loss in the 20th and 21st Centuries," PR Newswire Research and Markets, August 13, 2021, prnewswire.com/news-releases/global-weight-loss-products-and-services-market-report-2021-the-business-of-weight-loss-in-the-20th-and-21st-centuries-301354957.html.

3. "Is Red Meat Bad for You?," Cleveland Clinic Health Essentials, December 22, 2020, health.clevelandclinic.org/is-red-meat-bad-for-you.

4. L. Gianini et al., "Abnormal eating behavior in video-recorded meals in anorexia nervosa," *Eating Behaviors* 19 (December 2015): 28–32.

5. L. Birmingham et al., *Medical Management of Eating Disorders: A Practical Handbook for Healthcare Providers* (Cambridge, UK: Cambridge University Press, 2010).

6. J. Yager et al., *Practice Guideline for the Treatment of Patients with Eating Disorders* (Washington, DC: American Psychiatric Association, 2000): 1–39.

7. L. Belak et al., "Measurement of fidgeting in patients with anorexia nervosa using a novel shoe-based monitor," *Eating Behavior* 24 (January 2017): 45–48.

8. M. J. De Souza et al., "Expert Panel: 2014 Female Athlete Triad Coalition Consensus Statement on Treatment and Return to Play of the Female Athlete Triad: 1st International Conference held in San Francisco, California, May 2012 and 2nd International Conference held in Indianapolis, Indiana, May 2013," *British Journal of Sports Medicine* 48, no. 4 (February 2014): 289.

9. J. Berry, "What is 'morning wood,' and why does it happen?," Medical News Today, May 29, 2019, medicalnewstoday.com/articles/325305.

10. L. J. Goldberg and Y. Lenzy, "Nutrition and hair," *Clinics in Dermatology* 28, no. 4 (July–August 2010): 412–19.

    "The Best Vitamins and Supplements for Hair Growth," Cleveland Clinic Health Essentials, August 12, 2022, health.clevelandclinic.org/the-best-vitamins-supplements-and-products-for-healthier-hair.

11. J. L. Scheid and M. E. Stefanik, "Drive for Thinness Predicts Musculoskeletal Injuries in Division II NCAA Female Athletes," *Journal of Functional Morphology and Kinesiology* 4, no. 3 (August 2019): 52.

    J. M. Thein-Nissenbaum et al., "Associations Between Disordered Eating, Menstrual Dysfunction, and Musculoskeletal Injury Among High School Athletes," *Journal of Orthopaedic & Sports Physical Therapy* 41, no. 2 (February 2011): 42–119.

    J. J. Thomas et al., "Disordered eating and injuries among adolescent ballet dancers," *Eating and Weight Disorders - Studies on Anorexia, Bulimia and Obesity* 16, no. 3 (September 2011): e216–22.

12. S. Naessen et al., "Bone mineral density in bulimic women – influence of endocrine factors and previous anorexia," *European Journal of Endocrinology* 155, no. 2 (August 2006): 245–51.

13. L. Almeida, "What Is Body Checking?," Verywell Mind, March 22, 2022, verywellmind.com/reduce-body-checking-with-two-easy-steps-1138366.

Chapter 3

1. A. Nehlig, "Interindividual Differences in Caffeine Metabolism and Factors Driving Caffeine Consumption," *Pharmacological Reviews* 70, no. 2 (April 2018): 384–411.

2. R. L. Bailey et al., "Estimating caffeine intake from energy drinks and dietary supplements in the United States," *Nutrition Reviews* 72, suppl. 1 (October 2014): 9–13.

3. K. A. Wickham and L. L. Spriet, "Administration of caffeine in alternate forms," *Sports Medicine* 48, suppl. 1 (March 2018): 79–91.

4. R. J. Maughan and J. Griffin, "Caffeine ingestion and fluid balance: a review," *Journal of Human Nutrition and Dietetics* 16, no. 6 (December 2003): 411–20.

S. C. Killer et al., "No evidence of dehydration with moderate daily coffee intake: a counterbalanced cross-over study in a free-living population," *PloS One* 9, no. 1 (January 2014): e84154.

Y. Zhang et al., "Caffeine and diuresis during rest and exercise: a meta-analysis," *Journal of Science and Medicine in Sport* 18, no. 5 (2015): 569–74.

5. J. Johnson, "How long does a cup of coffee keep you awake?," Medical News Today, May 13, 2018, medicalnewstoday.com/articles/321784.

B. E. Statland and T. J. Demas, "Serum caffeine half-lives. Healthy subjects vs. patients having alcoholic hepatic disease," *American Journal of Clinical Pathology* 73, no. 3 (March 1980): 390–93.

N. S. Guest et al., "International society of sports nutrition position stand: caffeine and exercise performance," *Journal of the International Society of Sports Nutrition* 18, no. 1 (2021): 1.

6. D. A. Klein et al., "Intake, sweetness and liking during modified sham feeding of sucrose solutions," *Physiology & Behavior* 87, no. 3 (2006): 602–6.

T. A. Brown and P. K. Keel, "What contributes to excessive diet soda intake in eating disorders: appetitive drive, weights concerns, or both?," *Eating Disorders* 21, no. 3 (April 2013): 265–74.

D. A. Klein et al., "Artificial sweetener use among individuals with eating disorders," *International Journal of Eating Disorders* 39, no. 4 (May 2006): 341–45.

7. C. M. Shapiro, "Sleep and the athlete," *British Journal of Sports Medicine* 15, no. 1 (March 1981): 51–55.

D. A. Cohen et al., "Uncovering residual effects of chronic sleep loss on human performance," *Science Translational Medicine* 2, no. 14 (January 2010):14ra3.

8. C. D. Mah et al., "The Effects of Sleep Extension on the Athletic Performance of Collegiate Basketball Players," *Sleep* 34, no. 7 (July 2011): 943–50.

9. M. D. Milewski et al., "Chronic lack of sleep is associated with increased sports injuries in adolescent athletes," *Journal of Pediatric Orthopaedics* 34, no. 2 (March 2014): 129–33.

10. "How Optimizing Sleep Optimizes Well-Being," Therapy Rocks!, March 28, 2021, audio, audioboom.com/posts/7832530-how-optimizing-sleep-optimizes-well-being.

Chapter 4

1. N. H. Golden et al., "Higher caloric intake in hospitalized adolescents with anorexia nervosa is associated with reduced length of stay and no increased rate of refeeding syndrome," *Journal of Adolescent Health* 53, no. 5 (November 2013): 573–78.

2. S. F. Forman et al., "An eleven site national quality improvement evaluation of adolescent medicine-based eating disorder programs: Predictors of weight outcomes at one year and risk adjustment analyses," *Journal of Adolescent Health* 49, no. 6 (December 2011): 594–600.

3. "What is Misophonia?," soQuiet, soquiet.org/whatismisophonia.

Chapter 5

1. J. Slavin and J. Carlson, "Carbohydrates," *Advances in Nutrition* 5, no. 6 (November 2014): 760–61.

2. "Gluten Intolerance," Cleveland Clinic, last modified June 30, 2021, my.clevelandclinic.org/health/diseases/21622-gluten-intolerance.

3. "About NSF," National Sanitation Foundation, nsf.org/about-nsf.

4. "Dietary Supplement Manufacturing – UPS Verified Mark," United States Pharmacopeial Convention, usp.org/verification-services/verified-mark.

    "Certified Dietary Supplements," Informed Choice, choice.wetestyoutrust.com.

5. S. Egan, "How Much Protein Do We Need?," *The New York Times*, July 28, 2017.

6. D. McDonald et al., "American Gut: an Open Platform for Citizen Science Microbiome Research," *mSystems* 3, no. 3 (May 2018): e00031–18.

7. C.-Y. Chang et al., "Essential fatty acids and human brain," *Acta Neurologica Taiwanica* 18, no. 4 (December 2009): 231–41.

8. J. H. Davies et al., "Bone mass acquisition in healthy children," *Disease in Childhood* 90, no. 4 (March 2005): 373–78.

9. M.-X. Ji and Q. Yu, "Primary osteoporosis in postmenopausal women," *Chronic Diseases and Translational Medicine* 1, no. 1 (March 2015): 9–13.

10. "Menopause and Bone Loss," Endocrine Society, January 24, 2022, endocrine.org/patient-engagement/endocrine-library/menopause-and-bone-loss.

Chapter 6

1. B. Kochavi et al., "Resting energy expenditure in acutely ill and stabilized patients with anorexia nervosa and bulimia nervosa," *International Journal of Eating Disorders* 53, no. 9 (September 2020): 1460–68.

    N. Vaisman et al., "Energy expenditure and body composition in patients with anorexia nervosa," *Journal of Pediatrics* 113, no. 5 (November 1988): 919–24.

    D. D. Krahn et al., "Changes in resting energy expenditure and body composition in anorexia nervosa patients during refeeding," *Journal of the American Dietetic Association* 93, no. 4 (April 1993): 434–38.

    J. E. Schebendach et al., "The metabolic responses to starvation and refeeding in adolescents with anorexia nervosa," *Annals of the New York Academy of Sciences* 817 (May 1997): 110–19.

2. W. Kaye et al., "Caloric intake necessary for weight maintenance in anorexia nervosa: nonbulimics require greater caloric intake than bulimics," *American Journal of Clinical Nutrition* 44, no. 4 (October 1986): 435–43.

    J. Walker et al., "Caloric requirements for weight gain in anorexia nervosa," *American Journal of Clinical Nutrition* 32, no. 7 (July 1979): 1396–1400.

3. J. E. Schebendach et al., 1997, op. cit.

4. N. H. Golden and W. Meyer, "Nutritional Rehabilitation of Anorexia Nervosa. Goals and Dangers," *International Journal of Adolescent Medicine and Health* 16, no. 2 (April–June 2004): 131–44.

    J. Yager et al., *Practice Guideline for the Treatment of Patients with Eating Disorders* (Washington, DC: American Psychiatric Association, 2000): 1–39.

5. N. H. Golden et al., "Higher caloric intake in hospitalized adolescents with anorexia nervosa is associated with reduced length of stay and no increased rate of refeeding syndrome," *Journal of Adolescent Health* 53, no. 5 (November 2013): 573–78; see also D. Le Grange et al., "Early weight gain predicts outcome in two treatments for adolescent anorexia nervosa," *International Journal of Eating Disorders* 47, no. 2 (March 2014): 124–29.

    C. Crone et al., *Practice Guideline for the Treatment of Patients with Eating Disorders*, 4th Edition (Washington, DC: American Psychiatric Association, 2023): 167–71.

Chapter 9

1. E. A. Olansson et al., "Small particle size diet reduces upper gastrointestinal symptoms in patients with diabetic gastroparesis: a randomized controlled trial," *American Journal of Gastroenterology* 109, no. 3 (March 2014): 375–85.

2. J. E. Schebendach et al., "The metabolic responses to starvation and refeeding in adolescents with anorexia nervosa," *Annals of the New York Academy of Sciences* 817 (May 1997): 110–19.

3. C. P. Ferguson et al., "Are serotonin selective reuptake inhibitors effective in underweight anorexia nervosa?," *International Journal of Eating Disorders* 25, no. 1 (January 1999): 11–17.

   W. H. Kaye et al., "Neurobiology of anorexia nervosa: clinical implications of alterations of the function of serotonin and other neuronal systems," *International Journal of Eating Disorders* 37, suppl. (2005): S15–19.

4. A. Sifferlin, "Why You Might Want to Start Taking Fish Oil," Time, April 26, 2016.

5. I. Lete and J. Allué, "The Effectiveness of Ginger in the Prevention of Nausea and Vomiting during Pregnancy and Chemotherapy," *Integrative Medicine Insights* 11 (March 2016): 11–17.

6. M. L. Hu et al., "Effect of ginger on gastric motility and symptoms of functional dyspepsia," *World Journal of Gastroenterology* 17, no. 1 (January 2011): 105–10.

7. C. Mohr et al., "Peppermint Essential Oil for Nausea and Vomiting in Hospitalized Patients: Incorporating Holistic Patient Decision Making into the Research Design," *Journal of Holistic Nursing* 39, no. 2 (June 2021): 126–34.

   M. Maghami et al., "The effect of aromatherapy with peppermint essential oil on nausea and vomiting after cardiac surgery: A randomized clinical trial," *Complementary Therapies in Clinical Practice* 40 (August 2020): 101199.

   M. Karsten et al., "Effects of Peppermint Aromatherapy on Postoperative Nausea and Vomiting," *Journal of PeriAnesthesia Nursing* 35, no. 6 (December 2020): 615–18.

8. B. Ottillinger et al., "STW 5 (Iberogast®)—a safe and effective standard in the treatment of functional gastrointestinal disorders," *Wiener Medizinische Wochenschrift* 163, no. 3–4 (February 2013): 65–72.

9. P. Westmoreland et al., "Medical Complications of Anorexia Nervosa and Bulimia," *American Journal of Medicine* 129, no. 1 (January 2016): 30–37.

10. "Controlling Intestinal Gas," International Foundation for Gastrointestinal Disorders, iffgd.org/gi-disorders/symptoms-causes/intestinal-gas.

11. G. T. Doran, "There's a S.M.A.R.T. Way to Write Management's Goals and Objectives," *Management Review* 70 (1981): 35–36.

Chapter 10

1. L. Brelet et al., "Stigmatization toward People with Anorexia Nervosa, Bulimia Nervosa, and Binge Eating Disorder: A Scoping Review," *Nutrients* 13, no. 8 (August 2021): 2834.

    E. S. Rome and S. Ammerman, "Medical complications of eating disorders: An update," *Journal of Adolescent Health* 33 (December 2003): 418–26.

    L. M. Hart et al., "Unmet need for treatment in the eating disorders: A systematic review of eating disorder specific treatment seeking among community cases," *Clinical Psychology Review* 31, no. 5 (July 2011): 727–35.

2. J. Arcelus et al., "Mortality rates in patients with anorexia nervosa and other eating disorders: A meta-analysis of 36 studies," *Archives of General Psychiatry* 68, no. 7 (2011): 724–31.

3. R. J. Stanborough and M. Lee, "9 Tips for Finding the Right Therapist," Healthline, last modified April 28, 2023, healthline.com/health/how-to-find-a-therapist.

4. "Find a Health at Every Size® Healthcare Provider," Association for Size Diversity and Health, asdah.org/haes-professional.

Chapter 11

1. P. Shetty, "Malnutrition and undernutrition," *Medicine* 31, no. 4 (April 2003): 18–22.

2. P. S. Mehler and A. E. Andersen, *Eating Disorders: A Guide to Medical Care and Complications*, 2nd Edition (Baltimore, MD: Johns Hopkins University Press, 2010).

3. M. R. Kohn et al., "Cardiac arrest and delirium: presentations of the refeeding syndrome in severely malnourished adolescents with anorexia nervosa," Journal of Adolescent Health 22, no. 3 (March 1998): 239–43.

4. R. M. Ornstein et al., "Hypophosphatemia during nutritional rehabilitation in anorexia nervosa: implications for refeeding and monitoring," *Journal of Adolescent Health* 32, no. 1 (January 2003): 83–88.

S. M. Solomon and D. F. Kirby, "The refeeding syndrome: a review," *Journal of Parenteral and Enteral Nutrition* 14, no. 1 (January–February 1990): 90–97.

5. J. Yager et al., *Practice Guideline for the Treatment of Patients with Eating Disorders*, 3rd Edition (Washington, DC: American Psychiatric Association, 2010).

6. C. Crone et al., *Practice Guideline for the Treatment of Patients with Eating Disorders*, 4th Edition (Washington, DC: American Psychiatric Association, 2023): 167–71.

7. C. Wiklund, "Evaluating disorders of the gut-brain interaction in eating disorders," *International Journal of Eating Disorders* 54, no. 6 (June 2021): 925–35.

8. P. S. Mehler and A. E. Andersen, *Eating Disorders: A Guide to Medical Care and Complications*, 4th Edition (Baltimore, MD: Johns Hopkins University Press, 2022).

9. J. Baker, "The Role of Reproductive Hormones in the Development and Maintenance of Eating Disorders," *Expert Review of Obstetrics & Gynecology* 7, no. 6 (November 2012): 573–83.

10. Mehler and Andersen, 2010, op. cit.

11. A. Drabkin et al., "Assessment and clinical management of bone disease in adults with eating disorders: a review," *International Journal of Eating Disorders* 5 (2017): 42.

12. Practice Committee of the American Society for Reproductive Medicine, "Current Evaluation of Amenorrhea," *Fertility and Sterility* 86, no. 5, suppl. 1 (November 2006): S148–55.

13. Mehler and Andersen, 2010, op. cit.

14. Mehler and Andersen, 2022, op. cit.

15. M. S. Linna et al., "Reproductive health outcomes in eating disorders," *International Journal of Eating Disorders* 46, no. 8 (December 2013): 826–33.

16. A. Easter et al., "Recognising the symptoms: how common are eating disorders in pregnancy?," *European Eating Disorders Review* 21, no. 4 (July 2013): 340–44.

17. K. K. Kummer et al., "Aging male symptomatology and eating behavior," *The Aging Male* 22, no. 1 (March 2019): 55–61.

E. Midlarsky et al., "Eating Disorders in Middle-Aged Women," *Journal of General Psychology* 135, no. 4 (2008): 393–407.

18. Mehler and Andersen, 2022, op. cit.

19. S. Zipfel et al., "Osteoporosis and eating disorders: a follow-up study of patients with anorexia and bulimia nervosa," *Journal of Clinical Endocrinology and Metabolism* 86, no. 11 (November 2001): 5227–33.

20. Mehler and Andersen, 2010, op. cit.

21. Mehler and Andersen, 2022, op. cit.

22. P. K. Keel et al., "Predictors of Mortality in Eating Disorders," *Archives of General Psychiatry* 60, no. 2 (February 2003): 179–83.

23. K. Devlin, "Top 10 Reasons Why the BMI Is Bogus," Weekend Edition Saturday, July 4, 2009, npr.org/templates/story/story.php?storyId=106268439.

24. Ibid.

25. L. M. Brownstone et al., "Dismantling weight stigma: A group intervention in a partial hospitalization and intensive outpatient eating disorder treatment program," *Psychotherapy* 58, no. 2 (June 2021): 282–87.

26. T. L. Tylka et al., "The weight-inclusive versus weight-normative approach to health: Evaluating the evidence for prioritizing well-being over weight loss," Journal of Obesity 2014 (July 2014).

27. A. Goodwin, "'Don't Weigh Me' cards aim to reduce stress at the doctor's office," CNN Health, December 22, 2021, cnn.com/2021/12/22/health/dont-weigh-me-cards-wellness/index.html.

28. "Eating Disorder Guide for Parents," more-love.org.

29. E. M. Matheson et al., "Healthy Lifestyle Habits and Mortality in Overweight and Obese Individuals," *Journal of the American Board of Family Medicine* 25, no. 1 (January 2012): 9–15.

30. S. Bangalore et al., "Body-Weight Fluctuations and Outcomes in Coronary Disease," *New England Journal of Medicine* 376, no. 14 (April 2017): 1332–40.

31. L. M. Brownstone et al., 2021, op. cit.

32. A. F. Ralph et al., "Management of eating disorders for people with higher weight: clinical practice guideline," *International Journal of Eating Disorders* 10, no. 1 (August 2022): 121.

33. T. L. Tylka et al., 2014, op. cit.

Chapter 12

1. E. Vall and T. D. Wade, "Predictors of treatment outcome in individuals with eating disorders: A systematic review and meta-analysis," *International Journal of Eating Disorders* 48, no. 7 (July 2015): 946–71.

2. A. Lafrance et al., *Emotion-Focused Family Therapy: A Transdiagnostic Model for Caregiver-Focused Interventions* (Washington, DC: American Psychological Association, 2020).

3. J. O. Prochaska and C. C. DiClemente, "Toward a comprehensive model of change," in W. R. Miller and N. Heather, eds., *Treating Addictive Behaviors: Processes of Change* (New York: Springer, 1986), 3–27.

4. E. Y. Chen et al., "A Case Series of Family-Based Therapy for Weight Restoration in Young Adults with Anorexia Nervosa," *Journal of Contemporary Psychotherapy* 40, no. 4 (December 2010): 219–24.

5. E. Y. Chen et al., "Family-Based Therapy for Young Adults with Anorexia Nervosa Restores Weight," *International Journal of Eating Disorders* 49, no. 7 (July 2016): 701–7.

6. Ibid.

7. S. Mulkens and G. Waller, "New developments in cognitive-behavioural therapy for eating disorders (CBT-ED)," *Current Opinion in Psychiatry* 34, no. 6 (November 2021): 576–83.

   P. Hay, "Current approach to eating disorders: a clinical update," *Internal Medicine Journal* 50, no. 1 (January 2020): 24–29.

8. R. Murphy et al., "Cognitive Behavioral Therapy for Eating Disorders," *Psychiatric Clinics of North America* 33, no. 3 (September 2010): 611–27.

9. A. S. Lenz et al., "Effectiveness of Dialectical Behavior Therapy for Treating Eating Disorders," *Journal of Counseling & Development* 92, no. 1 (January 2014): 26–35.

   D. Ben-Porath et al., "Dialectical behavioral therapy: an update and review of the existing treatment models adapted for adults with eating disorders," *International Journal of Eating Disorders* 28, no. 2 (March–April 2020): 101–21.

10. S. M. Bankoff et al., "A systematic review of dialectical behavior therapy for the treatment of eating disorders," *International Journal of Eating Disorders* 20, no. 3 (2012): 196–215.

11. T. R. Lynch et al., "Radically open-dialectical behavior therapy for adult anorexia nervosa: feasibility and outcomes from an inpatient program," *BMC Psychiatry* 13, no. 293 (2013).

12. Ibid.

13. R. Harris, *The Happiness Trap: How to Stop Struggling and Start Living*, 2nd Edition (Boulder, CO: Shambhala Publications, 2022).

14. R. Grenon et al., "Group psychotherapy for eating disorders: A meta-analysis," *International Journal of Eating Disorders* 50, no. 9 (September 2017): 997–1013.

15. S. Neufeld, "Yoga Therapy, Asking for Help, and Avoiding the 'All Natural' Mandate," Therapy Rocks!, January 14, 2022, audio, audioboom.com/posts/8013305-yoga-therapy-asking-for-help-and-avoiding-the-all-natural-mandate.

Chapter 13

1. J. Sundgot-Borgen and M. K. Torstveit, "Prevalence of Eating Disorders in Elite Athletes Is Higher Than in the General Population," *Clinical Journal of Sport Medicine* 14, no. 1 (January 2004): 25–32.

2. M. Mountjoy et al., "The IOC consensus statement: beyond the Female Athlete Triad—Relative Energy Deficiency in Sport (RED-S)," *British Journal of Sports Medicine* 48, no.7 (March 2014): 491–97.

3. L. M. Burke et al., "Relative Energy Deficiency in Sport in Male Athletes: A Commentary on Its Presentation Among Selected Groups of Male Athletes," *International Journal of Sport Nutrition and Exercise Metabolism* 28, no. 4 (July 2018): 364–74.

4. B. W. Fudge et al., "Evidence of negative energy balance using doubly labelled water in elite Kenyan endurance runners prior to competition," *British Journal of Nutrition* 95, no. 1 (January 2006): 59–66.

5. E. N. Muia et al., "Adolescent elite Kenyan runners are at risk for energy deficiency, menstrual dysfunction and disordered eating," *Journal of Sports Sciences* 34, no. 7 (2016): 598–606.

    L.M. Burke et al., 2018, op. cit.

6. C. A. Dueck et al., "Treatment of athletic amenorrhea with a diet and training intervention program," *International Journal of Sport Nutrition and Exercise Metabolism* 6, no. 1 (March 1996): 24–40.

7. I. L. Fahrenholtz et al., "Within-day energy deficiency and reproductive function in female endurance athletes," *Scandinavian Journal of Medicine & Science in Sports* 28, no. 3 (March 2018): 1139–46.

8. G. Mastorakos et al., "Exercise and the stress system," *Hormones (Athens)* 4, no. 2 (April–June 2005): 73–89.

    N. J. Rinaldi et al., *No Period. Now What?: A Guide to Regaining Your Cycles and Improving Your Fertility* (Antica Press LLC, 2016).

9. M. Freimuth et al., "Clarifying exercise addiction: Differential diagnosis, co-occurring disorders, and phases of addiction," *International Journal of Environmental Research and Public Health* 8, no. 10 (October 2011): 4069–81.

10. J. Carter et al., "Relapse in anorexia nervosa: A survival analysis," *Psychological Medicine* 34, no. 4 (May 2004): 671–79.

    M. Strober et al., "The long-term course of severe anorexia nervosa in adolescents: Survival analysis of recovery, relapse, and outcome predictors over 10–15 years in a prospective study," *International Journal of Eating Disorders* 22, no. 4 (December 1997): 339–60.

    R. D. Grave et al., "Compulsive exercise to control shape or weight in eating disorders: prevalence, associated features, and treatment outcome," *Comprehensive Psychiatry* 49, no. 4 (July-August 2008): 346–52.

11. D. Godoy-Izquierdo et al., "A Systematic Review on Exercise Addiction and the Disordered Eating-Eating Disorders Continuum in the Competitive Sport Context," *International Journal of Mental Health and Addiction* 21 (August 2021): 529–61.

12. J. A. Martenstyn et al., "Treatment Considerations for Compulsive Exercise in High-Performance Athletes with an Eating Disorder," *Sports Medicine - Open* 8, no. 1 (March 2022): 30.

13. Ibid.

14. J. A. Martenstyn et al., "Treatment of compulsive exercise in eating disorders and muscle dysmorphia: protocol for a systematic review," *Journal of Eating Disorders* 9, no. 1 (February 2021): 19.

15. C. Law and C. L. Boisseau, "Exposure and response prevention in the treatment of obsessive-compulsive disorder: current perspectives," *Psychology Research and Behavior Management* 12 (2019): 1167–74.

16. B. D. Sylvester et al., "Variety support and exercise adherence behavior: experimental and mediating effects," *Journal of Behavioral Medicine* 39, no. 2 (April 2016): 214–24.

    N. M. Glaros and C. M. Janelle, "Varying the mode of cardiovascular exercise to increase adherence," *Journal of Sport Behavior* 24, no. 1 (2001): 42–62.

17. J. A. Martenstyn et al., 2021, op. cit.

18. O. Walker, "Heart Rate Variability (HRV)," *Science for Sport*, January 27, 2017, scienceforsport.com/heart-rate-variability-hrv.

Chapter 14

1. M. Galbally et al., "Management of anorexia nervosa in pregnancy: a systematic and state-of-the-art review," *Lancet Psychiatry* 9, no. 5 (May 2022): 402–12.

2. P. Westmoreland et al., "Medical Complications of Anorexia Nervosa and Bulimia," *American Journal of Medicine* 129, no. 1 (January 2016): 30–37.

    S. Koubaa et al., "Pregnancy and neonatal outcomes in women with eating disorders," *Obstetrics & Gynecology* 105, no. 2 (February 2005): 255–60.

    M. G. Katz and B. Vollenhoven, "The reproductive endocrine consequences of anorexia nervosa," *BJOG* 107, no. 6 (June 2000): 707–13.

3. R. L. Naeye, "Weight gain and the outcome of pregnancy," *American Journal of Obstetrics and Gynecology* 135, no. 1 (September 1979): 3–9.

4. N. Micali et al., "Fertility Treatment, Twin Births, and Unplanned Pregnancies in Women with Eating Disorders: Findings from a Population-Based Birth Cohort," *BJOG* 121, no. 4 (March 2014): 408–16.

5. G. J. Cuskelly et al., "Effect of increasing dietary folate on red-cell folate: implications for prevention of neural tube defects," *Lancet* 347, no. 9002 (1996): 657–59.

6. J. Stephenson et al., "Before the beginning: nutrition and lifestyle in the preconception period and its importance for future health," *Lancet* 391, no. 10132 (May 2018): 1830–41.

7. C. A. Rosenbloom and E. Coleman, "Pregnancy and Exercise," in C. Karpinski and C. A. Rosenbloom (eds.), *Sports Nutrition: A Practice Manual for Professionals* (Chicago: Academy of Nutrition and Dietetics, 2012).

8. "Weight Gain During Pregnancy," Centers for Disease Control and Prevention, last modified June 13, 2022, cdc.gov/reproductivehealth/maternalinfanthealth/pregnancy-weight-gain.htm.

9. M. Galbally et al., 2022, op. cit.

10. M. A. Kominiarek and P. Rajan, "Nutrition Recommendations in Pregnancy and Lactation," *Medical Clinics of North America* 100, no. 6 (November 2016): 1199–1215.

11. "How much water should I drink during pregnancy?," Ask ACOG: The American College of Obstetricians and Gynecologists, last modified October 2020, acog.org/womens-health/experts-and-stories/ask-acog.

"Nursing Your Baby: What You Eat and Drink Matters," Eat Right, last modified March 28, 2022, eatright.org/health/pregnancy/breastfeeding-and-formula/nursing-your-baby-what-you-eat-and-drink-matters.

12. J. J. Otten et al. (eds.), *Dietary Reference Intakes: The Essential Guide to Nutrient Requirements* (Washington, DC: National Academies Press, 2006).

13. F. P. McCarthy et al., "Hyperemesis gravidarum: current perspectives," *International Journal of Women's Health* 6 (2014): 719–25.

14. I. Lete and J. Allué, "The Effectiveness of Ginger in the Prevention of Nausea and Vomiting during Pregnancy and Chemotherapy," *Integrative Medicine Insights* 11 (March 2016): 11–17.

15. "Pregnancy and Heartburn," Stanford Medicine: Children's Health, stanfordchildrens.org/en/topic/default?id=pregnancy-and-heartburn-134-10.

16. L. Nichols, *Real Food for Pregnancy: The Science and Wisdom of Optimal Prenatal Nutrition* (self-published, 2018).

17. P. Westmoreland et al., 2016, op. cit.

18. "Gestational Diabetes - Symptoms, Treatments," American Diabetes Association, diabetes.org/diabetes/gestational-diabetes.

19. "Preeclampsia - Symptoms and causes," Mayo Clinic, August 15, 2022, mayoclinic.org/diseases-conditions/preeclampsia/symptoms-causes/syc-20355745.

20. K. Asayama and Y. Imai, "The impact of salt intake during and after pregnancy," *Hypertension Research* 41, no. 1 (January 2018): 1–5.

L. Nichols, 2018, op. cit.

21. V. Berghella and G. Saccone, "Exercise in pregnancy!," *American Journal of Obstetrics and Gynecology* 216, no. 4 (April 2017): 335–37.

D. Kolomanska-Boguck and A. I. Mazur-Bialy, "Physical Activity and the Occurrence of Postnatal Depression - A Systematic Review," *Medicina* (Kaunas) 55, no. 9 (September 2019): 560.

A. Nakamura et al., "Physical activity during pregnancy and postpartum depression: Systematic review and meta-analysis," *Journal of Affective Disorders* 246 (March 2019): 29–41.

22. M. K. Campbell and M. F. Mottola, "Recreational exercise and occupational activity during pregnancy and birth weight: a case-control study,"

American Journal of Obstetrics and Gynecology 184, no. 3 (February 2001): 403–8.

23. H. N. Soultanakis et al., "Prolonged exercise in pregnancy: glucose homeostasis, ventilatory and cardiovascular responses," *Seminars in Perinatology* 20, no. 4 (August 1996): 315–27.

    H. Syed et al., "ACOG Committee Opinion No. 804: Physical Activity and Exercise During Pregnancy and the Postpartum Period," *Obstetrics & Gynecology* 137, no. 2 (February 2021): 375–76.

24. Ibid.

25. "Nursing Your Baby: What You Eat and Drink Matters," 2022, op. cit.

26. M. E. Harrison et al., "Systematic review of the effects of family meal frequency on psychosocial outcomes in youth," *Canadian Family Physician* 61, no. 2 (February 2015): e96–106.

27. A. Bye et al., "Prevalence and clinical characterisation of pregnant women with eating disorders," *European Eating Disorder Review* 28, no. 2 (March 2020): 141–55.

28. S. Aggarwal et al., *Raising Body Positive Teens: A Parent's Guide to Diet-Free Living, Exercise and Body Image* (London: Jessica Kingsley Publishers, 2022).

29. J. A. Lydecker et al., "Associations of parents' self, child, and other 'fat talk' with child eating behaviors and weight," *International Journal of Eating Disorders* 51, no. 6 (June 2018): 527–34.

Chapter 16

1. L. L. Birch et al., "What Kind of Exposure Reduces Children's Food Neophobia?," *Appetite* 9, no. 3 (December 1987): 171–78; see also L. L. Birch and D. W. Marlin, "I Don't Like It; I Never Tried It: Effects of Exposure on Two-Year-Old Children's Food Preferences," *Appetite* 3, no. 4 (December 1982): 353–60.

Chapter 18

1. "The $72 Billion Weight Loss & Diet Control Market in the United States, 2019–2023 - Why Meal Replacements are Still Booming, but Not OTC Diet Pills - ResearchAndMarkets.com," *Business Wire*, February 25, 2019.

    "How Much Is the Beauty Industry Worth? (2015–2027)," Oberlo, oberlo.com/statistics/how-much-is-the-beauty-industry-worth.

2. K. J. Homan and T. L. Tylka, "Development and exploration of the gratitude model of body appreciation in women," *Body Image* 25 (June 2018): 14–22.

R. Emmons, "What Gratitude Is Good," Greater Good magazine, November 16, 2010.

3. D. Carpenter, "The Science Behind Gratitude (and How It Can Change Your Life)," Happify, happify.com/hd/the-science-behind-gratitude.

4. S. L. Zaitsoff et al., "A longitudinal examination of body-checking behaviors and eating disorder pathology in a community sample of adolescent males and females," *International Journal of Eating Disorders* 53, no. 11 (November 2020): 1836–43.

5. J. E. Steinglass et al., "Targeting habits in anorexia nervosa: a proof-of-concept randomized trial," *Psychological Medicine* 48, no. 15 (November 2018): 2584–91.

6. K. Bernard, "Young People at 'Significant' Risk of Poor Body Image After Just Minutes on TikTok, Instagram, Researchers Say," *ABC News Australia*, September 29, 2022, abc.net.au/news/2022-09-29/tiktok-instagram-eating-disorders-research-griffith-university/101429038.

Chapter 20

1. "Adult Eating and Weight," Ellyn Satter Institute, ellynsatterinstitute.org/how-to-eat/adult-eating-and-weight.

2. N. H. Golden et al., "Resumption of menses in anorexia nervosa," *Archives of Pediatrics & Adolescent Medicine* 151, no. 1 (January 1997): 16–21.

3. S. Darpinian et al., *No Weigh!: A Teen's Guide to Positive Body Image, Food, and Emotional Wisdom* (London: Jessica Kingsley Publishers, 2018).

RESOURCES

Downloadable worksheets can be found at platebyplateapproach.com/all-products.

Eating Disorder Support Groups and Treatment Programs

Association for Size Diversity and Health (ASDAH): asdah.org

Body Reborn: bodyreborn.org

The Body Positive: thebodypositive.org

Eating Disorder Hope: eatingdisorderhope.com/recovery/support-groups

Eating Disorders Resource Center: edrcsv.org

Eating Disorder Referral & Information Center: edreferral.com/treatment

Equip (Telehealth for Eating Disorders): equip.health

FEDUP: A Trans+ & Intersex Collective: fedupcollective.org

The Garment Project: thegarmentproject.org

Liberating Jasper Virtual Support: liberatingjasper.com/supportgroups

Multi-Service Eating Disorders Association (MEDA): medainc.org/services/heal/get-help

National Alliance for Eating Disorders: allianceforeatingdisorders.com

Nalgona Positivity Pride: nalgonapositivitypride.com

Food Assistance Programs

Feeding America: feedingamerica.org

Meals on Wheels: mealsonwheelsamerica.org

Project HEAL: theprojectheal.org

US Department of Agriculture (USDA): usda.gov/topics/
food-and-nutrition

Hotlines

ANAD Helpline: 1-888-375-7767; anad.org

Postpartum Support International: 1-800-944-4773 (4PPD)

Suicide & Crisis Lifeline: 988

Further Reading on Eating Disorders and Body Image

Anti-Diet: Reclaim Your Time, Money, Well-Being, and Happiness Through Intuitive Eating, Christy Harrison MPH, RD

Awake at 3 a.m.: Yoga Therapy for Anxiety and Depression in Pregnancy and Early Motherhood, Suzannah Neufeld MFT, C-IAYT

The Body Is Not an Apology: The Power of Radical Self Love, 2nd Edition, Sonya Renee Taylor

Conquer Picky Eating for Teens and Adults: Activities and Strategies for Selective Eaters, Jenny McGlothlin, MS, SLP, and Katja Rowell, MD

Eating Disorders: A Comprehensive Guide to Medical Care and Complications, 4th edition, edited by Philip S. Mehler and Arnold E. Andersen

Eating Disorders: A Guide to Medical Care, 4th edition, Academy of Eating Disorders

Embody: Learning to Love Your Unique Body (and quiet that critical voice!), Connie Sobczak

Every Body Yoga: Let Go of Fear, Get On the Mat, Love Your Body, Jessamyn Stanley

Fat Talk: Parenting in the Age of Diet Culture, Virginia Sole-Smith

Fearing the Black Body: The Racial Origins of Fat Phobia, Sabrina Springs

How to Nourish Your Child Through an Eating Disorder, Casey Crosbie and Wendy Sterling

Learned Hopefulness: The Power of Positivity to Overcome Depression, Dan Tomasulo, PhD

No Weigh! A Teen's Guide to Positive Body Image, Food, and Emotional Wisdom, Signe Darpinian, Wendy Sterling, and Shelley Aggarwal

Pursuing Perfection: Eating Disorders, Body Myths, and Women at Midlife and Beyond, Margo Maine, PhD, FAED, CEDS, and Joe Kelly

Raising Body Positive Teens, Signe Darpinian, Wendy Sterling, and Shelley Aggarwal

The Recovery Mama Guide to Your Eating Disorder Recovery in Pregnancy and Postpartum, Linda Shanti McCabe

Self-Care 101: Self-Care Inspiration for Busy Parents, Kristi Yeh

Sick Enough: A Guide to Medical Complications of Eating Disorders, Jennifer Gaudiani

You Have the Right to Remain Fat, Virgie Tovar

Resources for People of Color

Finding a therapist

Black Mental Health Alliance: blackmentalhealth.com/connect-with-a-therapist

Choosing Therapy: choosingtherapy.com/finding-a-black-therapist

Melanin and Mental Health: melaninandmentalhealth.com

Therapy for Black Girls: providers.therapyforblackgirls.com

Therapy for Black Men: therapyforblackmen.org

Therapy for Latinx: therapyforlatinx.com

The Yellow Chair Collective (Asian American Therapy): yellowchaircollective.com

Mental health and general health care support

Health in Her Hue (Health Care Providers): healthinherhue.com

The National Asian American Pacific Islander Mental Health
Association: naapimha.org

Resources for the LGBTQIA+ Community

Fat and Queer: An Anthology of Queer and Trans Bodies and Lives,
edited by Bruce Owens Grimm, Miguel M. Morales, and Tiff Joshua
TJ Ferentini

Trevor Project: thetrevorproject.org

Relative Energy Deficiency in Sport (RED-S)

*Finding Your Sweet Spot: How to Avoid RED-S (Relative Energy Deficit
in Sport) by Optimizing Your Energy Balance*, Rebecca McConville

*No Period. Now What?: A Guide to Regaining Your Cycles and
Improving Your Fertility*, Dr. Nicola J Rinaldi, Stephanie G Buckler
Esq., Lisa Sanfilippo Waddell, illustrated by Mallory Blondin

Fun Table Games

Family Dinner Project: thefamilydinnerproject.org/fun/dinner-games

Numberless Scales

Blind Weight Scale: blindweight.com/products/blind-weight-scale

MyClearStep Scale: myclearstep.com

ACKNOWLEDGMENTS

We would like to thank Lesley Williams, MD, for saying yes and believing in this project—we are grateful for her weight-inclusive approach and her expertise in the field of eating disorders—she is a unicorn; Nan Shaw, LCSW, FBT, CEDS-S, for again joining us and sharing her wisdom with the world; Andrew Walen, LCSW-C, LICSW, CEDS-S, for sharing his lived experience as a male with an eating disorder; Suzannah Neufeld C-IAYT, CEDS-S for her expertise on yoga therapy; Riley Nickols, PhD, for his expertise in sports psychology and review of our exercise chapter; Danika Quesnel, MSc, for her guidance on dysfunctional movement; Kate Bennett, PsyD, Sport Psychologist, for graciously sharing her chart on mindful versus compulsive movement; Renee Urban, PT, Board Certified in Orthopedics, for her contribution on rest; Carrie Spindel, PsyD, for your review of our therapy chapter; Liz Dunn, MS, RD, LDN, for her guidance on athletes with disabilities; Lindsay Stenovec, MS, RD, CEDS-S, for her expert contributions on prenatal and postpartum wellness; Sarah Lowenthal, MD, CEDS-S, for her guidance on medications and nausea; Connie Sobczak, co-founder of The Body Positive, for her contributions on eating disorders and aging; and Sara Gilliam for her amazing edits and support early on! We are grateful to those who have been our cultural consultants and shared their delicious plates with us over the years, so we could share them with you. And lastly, we would like to thank all those fighting back against diet culture and weight stigma—without this fight, eating disorders will continue to exist.

To all the clients we have worked with over the years: Thank you for trusting us with your care. We are honored to be part of your journey. We are endlessly appreciative of our colleagues and mentors, who have been our teachers, friends, and support system through decades of work. We are grateful for the huge support we have received in the US and internationally for the Plate-by-Plate Approach®.

We would be remiss if we didn't mention those who personally supported and encouraged us from idea to publication. Wendy would like to thank her parents, Fran and Stuart Meyer, for their unconditional love and support. She thanks her daughters, Emily Sterling and Lexi Sterling, for their giggles, love, and amazing "picture plates." Finally, she would like to thank her husband, Peter Sterling, for always waiting just 2 more seconds to eat so she could take a picture, and also for his love, friendship, and unwavering support.

Casey would like to thank her family—her husband Ryan, for his endless support and interest in this work; her two young children, Maeve and Callum, who delight in eating and in observing the many differences of the human body; and to the baby she will meet just before this book is published, thank you for providing another lens from which to write about eating disorders in pregnancy—your timing was impeccable.

Last but not least, we would like to thank The Experiment for believing in us and for their commitment to the Plate-by-Plate Approach® and eating disorder recovery.

INDEX

A

AAN (atypical anorexia), 11–12

AAP (American Academy of Pediatrics), 9

accelerated nutritional rehabilitation
   for anorexia nervosa, 98, 100
   overview, 77–79
   plate breakdown and meal ideas, 80–84, 90–91
   sabotaging, 79–80

acceptance and commitment therapy (ACT), 168–69

acid reflux (heartburn), 200–1

acrocyanosis, 31, 145

ADHD (attention deficit hyperactivity disorder), 15

adolescence, 33

adolescent family-based therapy (FBT), 161–63

alcohol intake, 34, 117

almond milk, 75, 83

amenorrhea, 29, 31, 71, 140–41, 142–43, 192

American Academy of Pediatrics (AAP), 9

American Psychiatric Association (APA), 138; *see also* DSM-5

American Psychological Association, 128

angular cheilitis, 139, 145

anorexia nervosa (AN)
   case study, 98–100
   compensatory behaviors, 24
   diagnosis, 10, 11
   Plate-by-Plate Approach® for, 98–100

antacids, 115, 200

anxiety
   avoidant/restrictive food intake disorder and, 102, 103–4
   body checking behaviors and, 256
   comorbidity of eating disorders, 146
   eating disorder sign, 14, 34
   food fears, 214, 224–26; *see also* food fears
   muscle dysmorphia and, 14
   perinatal, 206–7

anxiety (*continued*)
    recovery and management
        of, 46
    sleep and, 45
    yoga therapy for, 171–72
APA (American Psychiatric
    Association), 138
appetizers, 82, 245
ARFID; *see* avoidant/restrictive
    food intake disorder
ASD (autism spectrum
    disorder), 15, 213
assessment
    baseline nutrition
        assessment, 38–45
    readiness assessment, 155–58
Association for Size Diversity
    and Health (ASDAH), 129
athletes, plate breakdown
    option, 49
attention deficit hyperactivity
    disorder (ADHD), 15
atypical anorexia (AAN), 11–12
autism spectrum disorder
    (ASD), 15, 213
avoidant/restrictive food intake
    disorder (ARFID); *see also*
    food fears
    case study, 101–4
    diagnosis, 11, 14–15
    Plate-by-Plate Approach® for,
        100–4
Awake at 3 a.m. (Neufield),
    171–72

B

"bad" foods (fear foods), 22, 127,
    208, 264
Barrett's esophagus, 139
barriers to Plate-by-Plate
    Approach®, 108–21
    appetite loss, 116–18
    gastrointestinal problems,
        109–16
    low energy and mood, 118–19
    motivation loss, 119–21
    overview, 108–9
    self-soothing options for, 121
baseline nutrition assessment,
    38–45
    diet assessment, 40–43
    food behaviors, 43–44
    food record, 39
    overview, 38, 45
    sleep assessment, 45
"bigorexia," 13–14
binge, defined, 12
binge eating disorder (BED)
    case study, 96–97, 149–50
    compensatory behaviors, 24
    diagnosis, 11, 12
    Plate-by-Plate Approach® for,
        95–97
bingeing, 21, 71, 144
BIPOC communities, 17, 149–
    50, 151–52, 305–6
birth control pills, 140–41
bloating/gas, 32, 109–10, 139

blood pressure levels, 135, 136, 203

blood sugar levels, 203

bluish discoloration of skin, 31, 145

BMD/DEXA scan, 144–45

BMI (body mass index), 146–47

BN; *see* bulimia nervosa

body checking, 14, 32, 256–57

body image dissatisfaction, 9, 20, 32–33, 143–44

The Body Positive Journal (Tovar), 251

body satisfaction, 250–60

    body checking reduction and, 256–57

    building a life outside of body identification, 259–60

    clothes shopping and, 254–56

    gratitude practice, 252–54

    overview, 250–51

    pausing for, 252

    self-weighing reduction and, 257–58

    separating feelings from food intake, 259

    social media and body dissatisfaction, 258–59

bone mass and bone health, 31, 73–74, 140, 141, 144–45

bradycardia (low heart rate), 29, 136

brain atrophy, 145–46

brain fog, 34

Bratman, Steven, 26

brittle nails, 30, 145

brown rice, 220

bulimia nervosa (BN)

    case study, 105–6

    diagnosis, 11, 12

    Plate-by-Plate Approach® for, 104–7

C

caffeine intake, 42–43, 117, 195

calcium, 72–74

carbohydrates, 62–64, 70, 220–21

cardiac irregularities, 29, 32, 135, 136, 137

CBT (cognitive behavioral therapy), 163–65, 166

CBT-E (enhanced cognitive behavioral therapy), 164

CBT-ED (cognitive behavioral therapy for EDs), 164

CDC (Centers for Disease Control and Prevention), 193–94

CEDRD (Certified Eating Disorder Registered Dietitian), 129

CEDS (Certified Eating Disorder Specialist), 126–27, 129

celiac disease, 8, 15, 64

Certified Specialist in Sports
    Dietetics (CSSD), 179
chest pain, 32, 137, 138
clean eating focus (orthorexia),
    26–27, 198
clothing, 254–56, 267–68
cognitive and psychological
    changes, 20, 33–34
cognitive behavioral therapy
    (CBT), 163–65, 166
cognitive behavioral therapy for
    EDs (CBT-ED), 164
cold intolerance, 31
communal meal avoidance, 24,
    33–34
complete blood count (CBC),
    141
comprehensive metabolic
    panel, 141
condiment use, 44
constipation, 112–13, 139, 201–2
Cortese, Kathy, 9
cravings, 95–96, 97, 200, 220–
    21, 273, 277
"crisis intervention" skills, 167
CSSD (Certified Specialist in
    Sports Dietetics), 179

D

dairy and dairy alternatives,
    72–76, 81, 83–84
dehydration, 32, 41, 42, 113, 141
delayed gastric emptying
    (gastroparesis), 109–10, 139
dental health, 144, 248–49
depression
    body checking behaviors and,
        256
    comorbidity of eating
        disorders, 146
    eating disorder sign, 14, 34
    hunger levels and, 277
    muscle dysmorphia and, 14
    perinatal, 206–7
    sleep and, 45
desserts, 82, 214, 245, 268
DEXA scan, 145
diabetes (gestational), 203
*Diagnostic and Statistical
    Manual of Mental Disorders,
    Fifth Edition* (DSM-5), 11–15
dialectical behavioral therapy
    (DBT), 165–68
diarrhea, 68, 139
diet; *see* baseline nutrition
    assessment
dieting, 3–4, 9, 21
dietitian, 126, 129–30, 179
disordered eating, 13, 18, 34,
    142–43
dissecting food, 25

distress tolerance skills, 166–67

dizziness, 28–29, 41

dry, plain food, 23

dry skin and hair, 30, 145

DSM-5 (*Diagnostic and Statistical Manual of Mental Disorders, Fifth Edition*), 11–15

dysfunctional movement, 27; *see also* exercise

E

eating behavior spectrum, 13, 24–25

eating disorders; *see also* exercise; medical issues
    age groups, 2, 9–11, 33, 143–44, 207–9
    defined, 13
    diagnosis, 11–15
    dieting and exchange systems, 3–4, 9, 21
    eating behavior spectrum, 13, 24–25
    in marginalized groups, 17–18, 149–50, 151–52, 305–6
    in men, 1, 15–16
    overview, 1–2, 8
    "recovery" from, 2–5; *see also* body satisfaction; navigating real life; normal eating;
        Plate-by-Plate Approach®; strategies for recovery
    resources on, 303–6
    what to look for, 19–34; *see also* signs and symptoms

ED Matters podcast, 9

EFAs (essential fatty acids), 71

electrolyte imbalances, 104, 137, 141, 146, 199

emotional loneliness, 168

endocrine (hormone) irregularities, 29–31, 33, 73–74, 139–140, 142, 179

eosinophilic esophagitis, 15

ERP (exposure and response prevention), 168, 182–83

essential fatty acids (EFAs), 71

estrogen levels, 29, 30–31, 71, 73–74

exchange systems (diet), 3–4

exercise, 173–89
    abstaining from, 187–88
    avoidance, 188–89
    behavior changes, 21, 27–28
    carbohydrates for, 63
    case study, 185
    closing the energy gap, 176–80
    compulsive, 180–85
    overview, 20, 27–28, 79–80, 173–74
    parenting advice, 208
    plate breakdown options for, 49, 50, 65

exercise (*continued*)
    during pregnancy, 202, 204–5
    relative energy deficiency in
        sport (RED-S), 174–76,
        306
    rest days, 178, 185–87
exposure and response
    prevention (ERP), 168, 182–83
exposure therapy, 2–3, 168–69,
    182–83, 213, 228–35

F

Fairburn, Christopher, 164
family and friends
    boundary-setting with, 264
    guidelines for, 261–70
    overview, 124–25, 132–33, 261
family-based therapy (FBT),
    161–63
famotidine, 112
fatigue, during pregnancy,
    202–3
fats, 69–72, 76, 83–84, 113
fear foods ("bad" foods), 22,
    208, 264
Female Athlete Triad, 175
fertility treatment, 192
fiber, 64, 102–3, 113, 115, 202
50% plate, 48–51, 77, 98, 100; *see
    also* accelerated nutritional
    rehabilitation

fine hair on face (lanugo),
    31–32, 145
fitness wearables (tracking
    devices), 183–84
folate and folic acid, 192–93
food assistance programs, 304
food combinations (abnormal),
    24–25
food fears
    baseline (pre-ED) favorite
        foods, 215, 223
    case studies, 230, 233–34
    eating in community, 215–16,
        223
    food rules, 216–22, 226–28
    overview, 2–3, 212–15
    varied diet and, 219–22
    vegetarian and vegan diets,
        217–18
food fears, strategies for
    step 1: knowing foods that
        escalate anxiety, 224–26
    step 2: fighting back against
        food rules, 226–28
    step 3 & 4: exposure, 228–35
food freedom; *see* body
    satisfaction; food fears;
    navigating real life; normal
    eating
food groups
    checklist, 52–53
    dairy and dairy alternatives,
        72–76, 81, 83–84
    fats, 69–72, 76, 83–84, 113

fruits and vegetables, 5, 31,
    67–69, 76
  grains and starches, 62–64,
    65, 66, 76, 219–20
  protein, 65–67, 76, 195–96
food insecurity, 176
food record, 39, 130
food rules, 216–22, 226–28
fractures, 30–31
friends and family; *see* family
  and friends
fruits and vegetables, 31, 67–69,
  76
fullness cues (satiety), 70–71,
  113–14, 116, 117, 242, 277–78

G

games, 306
gastroesophageal reflux disease
  (GERD), 139
gastrointestinal (GI) problems,
  15, 109–16, 138–39
gastroparesis (delayed gastric
  emptying), 109–10, 139
GBA (gut-brain axis), 138
gestational diabetes, 203
ginger, 111, 199, 201
gluten sensitivity, 52, 64–65,
  114–15, 216–17
goal-setting, 55–58
"good" foods, 22, 127, 208,
  221–22

grains and starches, 62–64, 65,
  66, 76, 219–20
gratitude practice, 252–54
group therapy, 170–71
gut-brain axis (GBA), 138
gynecologic/obstetric problems,
  140–41, 142–43; *see also*
  menopause; menstruation;
  pregnancy

H

hair issues, 30, 31–32, 145
headaches, 42, 204, 205
Health at Every Size® (HAES®),
  126–27
health consciousness, extreme
  (orthorexia), 26–27, 198
Health Food Junkies (Bratman),
  26
health messages, taken to the
  extreme, 22
"heaping half," 82
heartburn (acid reflux), 200–1
heart issues, 32, 135, 136, 137
heart rate, 29, 135, 136
heart rate variability (HRV)
  measurements, 183–84
hemorrhoids, 139, 201–2
high blood pressure
  (hypertension), 203
high blood sugar levels, 203
holiday meals, 244–45

hormone levels (endocrine irregularities), 29–31, 33, 73–74, 139–40, 142, 179

hotlines, 304

How to Nourish Your Child Through an Eating Disorder (Sterling & Crosbie), 2

hunger cues, 115–16, 117, 277–78

hydration, 41–42, 81, 112, 113, 196

hydroxyzine, 112

hypercarotemia (orange hands/ feet), 31, 68, 145

hyperprolactinemia, 140

hypertension (high blood pressure), 203

hypophosphatemia, 136–37

hypotension (low blood pressure), 135, 136

injuries and stress fractures, 30–31, 144–45

inner circle; *see* family and friends

inner circle support, 124–25, 132–33

Institute of Medicine (IOM), 62

International Association for Yoga Training (IAYT), 171

International Association of Eating Disorder Professionals (IAEDP), 126–27, 129

iron levels, 67

irritability, 34, 146

J

"jiggling," 251

Jones, Ginny, 148

I

IAEDP (International Association of Eating Disorders Professionals), 126–27, 129

IAYT (International Association for Yoga Training), 171

Iberogast, 111

infertility, 140, 142–43, 192

inflammatory bowel syndrome, 15

L

lab abnormalities, 141–42

lactase, 114–15

lactose intolerance, 74–75, 114–15

lanugo (fine hair on face), 31–32, 145

LGBTQ+ communities, 18, 151–52, 306

libido (sex drive), 29–30, 139, 144

Life Without Ed (Schaefer), 121, 154–55

Linehan, Marsha, 165

lipase, 114

lipid panel, 142

low blood pressure (hypotension), 135, 136

low energy and mood, 118–19

low resting heart rate (bradycardia), 29, 135

M

Maine, Margo, 9

malnutrition, 30–32, 41, 109–110, 134–37; *see also* medical issues

meals and meal ideas
    for accelerated rehabilitation, 90–91
    breakfast, 85–86
    for closing the energy gap, 176–77
    dinner, 88–89
    duration of, 57
    family guidelines on, 261–63
    goal-setting, 55
    lunch, 87–88
    normal eating guidelines, 278–80
    during pregnancy, 195–96
    scheduling, 57
    vegan plate, 91–92

medical issues
    cardiac irregularities, 29, 32, 135, 136, 137
    case study, 149–50
    dental/oral health, 144, 248–49
    dermatological symptoms, 145
    emergencies and urgent issues, 138
    endocrine (hormone) irregularities, 29–31, 33, 73–74, 139–40, 142, 179
    gastrointestinal problems, 15, 109–16, 138–39
    lab abnormalities, 141–42
    malnutrition, 30–32, 41, 109–10, 134–37
    in midlife, 143–44
    musculoskeletal symptoms, 144–45
    neurological symptoms, 34, 145–46
    obstetric/gynecological problems, 29, 31, 71, 140–41, 142–43, 192
    overview, 134
    psychiatric symptoms, 146
    seeking medical care, 147–48
    weight stigma, 146–47, 148, 150–51

medical support, 125–26, 128–29, 130–32, 147–51

medications, 130–31

menopause, 33, 73–74, 179

menstruation
cessation of (amenorrhea),
29, 31, 71, 140–41, 142–43,
192
irregularities, 140–41, 175,
179
oligomenorrhea, 29, 140, 192
perimenopause, 73–74, 179
messy eating, 25
metabolic panel, 141
metabolic recovery, 78–79, 110
metoclopramide, 112
midlife issues, 143–44
migraines, 146
milk, 73, 74–76, 81, 83–84, 244
milkshakes, 83
mindfulness, 182
mood changes, 34, 118, 146,
206–7; *see also* anxiety;
psychiatric symptoms
motivation loss, 119–21
mouth sores, 139
Musby, Eva, 161
muscle dysmorphia, 13–14
musculoskeletal symptoms,
144–45
must-attend events, 246
MyPlate (USDA), 4

N

nails (brittle), 30
nausea, 110–11, 139, 199
navigating real life, 236–49
holiday meals, 244–45
must-attend events, 246
overview, 236–37
religious dietary changes and
fasting, 245–46
restaurants, 237–41
sickness, 246–48
surgery and dental woes,
248–49
traveling, 242–44
work meals, 241–42
NEAT (non-exercise activity
thermogenesis), 28
nerve damage, 146
Neufeld, Suzannah, 171–72
neurological symptoms, 34,
145–46
Nickols, Riley, 179, 181, 184
nondairy milk, 75, 83, 220
non-exercise activity
thermogenesis (NEAT), 28
normal eating, 271–82
closing thoughts, 281–82
defined, 272–73
gaining confidence, 274–75
greater comfort around food,
275–76
hunger cues, 277–78
meal guidelines, 278–80
overview, 271–72

readiness for, 273–74

testing the waters, 276–77

trouble signs, 281

nutrition; *see* baseline nutrition assessment; malnutrition; Plate-by-Plate Approach®; registered dietitian

nutritional rehabilitation, 26

nutritional shakes, 82–83

O

obsessive thinking, 33

obstetric/gynecological problems, 140–41, 142–43; *see also* menopause; menstruation; pregnancy

oligomenorrhea, 29, 140, 192

omeprazole, 112

ondansetron, 112

one-pot meals, 53

optimized nutrition, 13

oral symptoms, 144

orange hands/feet (hypercarotemia), 31, 68, 145

orthorexia, 26–27, 198

orthostasis, 28–29, 135

orthostatic hypotension, 136

orthostatic tachycardia, 136

osteoporosis, 31, 73–74, 140, 144–45; *see also* bone mass and bone health

other specified feeding or eating disorder (OSFED), 11, 12–13, 24

oxalates, 73

P

pancreatic enzyme levels, 141–42

parenting, 190, 207–9

peppermint, 111, 112

perimenopause, 73–74, 179

peripheral neuropathy, 146

phosphorus levels, 136–37

physical activity; *see* exercise

pica, 11

pitting edema, 145

pizza, 241

plain, dry food, 23

Plan B Nutrition, 117–18

plant-based milk, 74–75, 83, 220

Plate-by-Plate Approach®

for accelerated nutritional rehabilitation, 77–84

for anorexia nervosa, 98–100

for avoidant/restrictive food intake disorder, 100–4

barriers to, 108–21; *see also* barriers to Plate-by-Plate Approach®

for binge eating disorder, 95–97

Plate-by-Plate Approach®
  (*continued*)
    breakdown of plate, 48–53,
      61–76, 80–84; *see also* food
      groups
    for bulimia nervosa, 104–7
    filling the plate, 53–55
    goal-setting, 55–58
    meal ideas, 85–92; *see also*
      meals and meal ideas
    nutrition assessment, 38–45;
      see also baseline nutrition
      assessment
    overview, 2, 4–5
    review of plate, 59–60
    selection of plate, 5
    size of plate, 46–48
    snack ideas, 92–94; *see also*
      snacks and snack ideas
polarizing foods, 208
polycystic ovarian syndrome,
  140
postpartum, 143, 190, 205–6
*Practice Guideline for the
  Treatment of Patients with
  Eating Disorders* (APA), 138
preeclampsia, 204
pre–esophageal cancer
  (Barrett's esophagus), 139
pregnancy, 190–209
    body image dissatisfaction
      and, 33
    before conception and
      infertility issues, 140,
      142–43, 191–93

constipation, 201–2
cravings, 200
definition, 190
exercise during, 202, 204–5
fatigue, 202–3
gestational diabetes, 203
heartburn, 200–1
hemorrhoids, 201–2
mood and anxiety disorders
  during, 206–7
nausea, 199
nutritional needs, 195–97
orthorexia during, 198
overview, 190–91
plate breakdown option, 49
postpartum, 143, 190, 205–6
preeclampsia, 204
as risk factor for eating
  disorders, 10–11
weight gain, 193–95
prenatal vitamins, 192–93, 197
protein, 65–67, 76, 195–96
protein powder, 66
psychiatric symptoms, 146; *see
  also* anxiety; depression
psychiatrists, 125, 126–28,
  130–31

Q

Quetelet, Lambert Adolphe
  Jacques, 146

R

radically open DBT (RO-DBT),
   167–68
Raynaud's phenomenon, 145
ready-to-drink supplement,
   82–83, 118
real life; *see* navigating real life
refeeding, 26, 114–15, 136–37
registered dietitian (RD), 126,
   129–30, 179
relative energy deficiency in
   sport (RED-S), 174–76, 306
religious dietary changes and
   fasting, 245–46
response prevention, 168
rest, from exercise, 178, 185–87
restaurants, 237–41
"reverse anorexia," 13–14
rice, 220
rice milk, 75
rigidity, as sign of eating
   disorder, 21
Ross, Kyra, 17
Rotach, Carise, 18
rules, as sign of eating disorder,
   21
rumination disorder, 11
Russell's sign, 145

S

"safe" foods, 221–22; *see also*
   "good" foods
Schaefer, Jenni, 121, 154–55
secondary amenorrhea, 140
seizures, 138, 146
self-care, 117, 133
self-soothing, 121
self-weighing, 257–58
seven-day food record, 39
sex drive (libido), 29–30, 139,
   144
shakes, 82–83
Shaw, Nan, 121
sickness, navigating in real life,
   246–48
signs and symptoms, 19–34
   body image issues, 32–33
   cognitive and psychological
      changes, 33–34
   exercise issues, 27–28
   food behavior changes, 21–27
   overview, 19–20, 34
   physical signs, 28–32
skin (dry), 30, 145
sleep, 43, 45, 144, 250
slow eating, 25
smoothies, 83, 244
snacks and snack ideas
   for accelerated nutritional
      rehabilitation, 81–82, 84
   for closing the energy gap,
      176–77
   defined, 56

snacks and snack ideas
(*continued*)
  duration of, 57
  goal-setting, 55–56
  overview, 92–94
  during pregnancy, 196
  scheduling, 57
Sobczak, Connie, 252
social eating avoidance, 24,
  33–34
social media, 258–59
spectrum of eating behavior, 13
spontaneity, lack of, 22–23
sports dietician, 179
starches and grains, 62–64, 65,
  66, 76, 219–20
Stice, E., 9
stigmas, 124–25, 146–47, 148,
  150–51
"straight, white, affluent girls"
  (SWAG), 18
strategies for recovery; *see also*
  Plate-by-Plate Approach®
    exposure process, 2–3, 168–
      69, 182–83, 213, 228–35
    inner circle support, 124–25,
      132–33
    medical, 125–26, 128–29,
      130–32, 138, 147–51
    nutritional, 126, 129–30, 179
    overview, 124–25
    therapy, 125, 126–28, 153–72
stress
  as barrier to recovery, 116–18
  exercise and, 178

stress fractures, 30–31, 144–45
supplements (ready-to-drink),
  82–83, 118
support
  inner circle, 124–25, 132–33
  medical, 125–26, 128–29,
    130–32, 147–51
  nutritionist, 126, 129–30, 179
  resources for support groups
    and programs, 303
  therapeutic strategies,
    125–28, 153–72; *see also*
    therapy
surgery, 248–49
SWAG ("straight, white, affluent
  girls"), 18
sweetener use, 44
sweet potatoes, 220

T

table behaviors, 25–26
table games, 306
testosterone levels, 29–31, 71,
  140, 175
therapy, 125–28, 153–72
  core tenets of, 158–60
  overview, 125, 126–28
  readiness assessment, 155–58
  resources, 303
  role in recovery, 153–55
  types of, 160–72
thinning hair, 30
33% plate, 48–49
Thompson, Ron, 179

thyroid panel, 142

Tovar, Virgie, 251

tracking devices (fitness wearables), 183–84

traveling, 242–44

treatment; *see* support

U

Urban, Renee, 185–86

urinalysis, 142

US Department of Agriculture (USDA), 4

V

vegetables and fruits, 31, 67–69, 76

vegetarian and vegan diets, 66–67, 74–75, 91–92, 217–18

vital signs, 135–36

vitamin D, 73, 74

vomiting, 138, 139

W

Walen, Andrew, 15–16

weight card, 148

weight changes (loss or gain)

exercise and, 178, 179–80

as physical sign of eating disorders, 28

during pregnancy, 193–94

weigh-ins at doctor's office, 148

weight gain difficulties, 77–79

weight-inclusive eating disorder management, 150–51

weight stigma, 146–47, 148, 150–51

white rice, 220

work meals, 241–42

X

xerosis (dry skin), 30, 145

Y

yoga therapy, 171–172

ABOUT THE AUTHORS

WENDY STERLING, MS, RD, CSSD, CEDS-S, specializes in eating disorders and sports nutrition. She has worked for the NFL, NBA, and MLB and is a frequent lecturer to schools and teams. She is the coauthor of *How to Nourish Your Child Through an Eating Disorder*, *Raising Body Positive Teens*, and *No Weigh!* Her work has also been published in the *International Journal of Eating Disorders*. She maintains a private practice in the San Francisco Bay Area.

CASEY CROSBIE, RD, CEDS-S, owns Crosbie Nutrition, a California-based private practice offering individual and family work as well as professional supervision and community outreach. She is the coauthor of *How to Nourish Your Child Through an Eating Disorder*. Her work has also been published in the *Journal of the Academy of Nutrition and Dietetics*. She lives in the Greater Sacramento area.

🅾 **platebyplateapproach**

ABOUT THE CONTRIBUTORS

LESLEY WILLIAMS, MD, is an eating disorder expert physician at Mayo Clinic in Scottsdale, Arizona. In addition to her family medicine practice, she is an advocate for weight inclusive care and author of the award-winning children's book, *Free to Be Me: Self Love for All Sizes*.

NAN SHAW, LCSW, FBT, CEDS-S, is an eating disorder and family therapy specialist, in private practice in the San Francisco Bay Area. She provides direct care as well as offering trainings, program development, parent coaching, and supervision.